Keto BBQ

SAUCES, RUBS, AND MARINADES

101 Low-Carb, Flavor-Packed Recipes
for Next-Level Grilling and Smoking

AILEEN ABLOG

This book is dedicated to everyone who is constantly building their best self.

***

Published in the U.S. by:
Ulysses Press
P. O. Box 3440
Berkeley, CA 94703
www.ulyssespress.com

ISBN: 978-1-64604-036-0
Library of Congress Control Number: 2020931868

Printed in the United States by Versa Press
10 9 8 7 6 5 4 3 2 1

Acquisitions editor: Casie Vogel
Managing editor: Claire Chun
Editor: Renee Rutledge
Proofreader: Kate St.Clair
Cover design: Leigh McDonald
Cover photograph: © Artim Shadrin/shutterstock.com
Interior design: what!design @ whatweb.com
Interior photos: © shutterstock.com; page 1 © nadianb; page 3 © Julia Sudnitskaya; page 8 © Nina Firsova; page 15 © Tatiana Volgutova; page 31 © nadianb; page 32 © a katz; page 33 © Elena Shashkina; page 34 © hlphoto; page 37 © Monkey Business Images; page 39 © Rebecca Fondren Photo; page 42 © a katz; page 43 © ACA9595; page 44 © Dewayne Flowers; page 46 © GPritchettPhoto; page 48 © stockcreations; page 50 © Africa Studio; page 52 © Indian Food Images; page 54 © Alexander Prokopenko; page 55 © encierro; page 56 © pamuk; page 59 © Stephanie Frey; page 61 © Elena Veselova; page 62 © Jacob Blount; page 63 © mama_mia; page 65 © Viktory Panchenko; page 66 © Aleksandrova Karina; page 67 © SMarina; page 71 © Oksana Mizina; page 72 © Matthew Scott 32; page 73 © from my point of view; page 79 © sasha2109; page 80 © MauricioSPY; page 81 © svariophoto; page 82 © etorres; pages 83, 113 © Brent Hofacker; page 85 © MaraZe; page 88 © bozulek; page 91 © Yulia Davidovich; page 93 © Andrey Starostin; page 94 © Anna Shepulova; pages 96, 108 © Elena Veselova; page 98 © rukxstockphoto; page 99 © thebeardandthebaker; page 103 © Alp Aksoy; page 104 © Humannet; page 106 © Indian Food Images; page 107 © Geshas; page 109 © Nickola Che; page 110 © Fascinadora; page 111 © Malisa Nicolau; page 115 © Vladimir VK; page 117 © Liliya Kandrashevich; page 118 © etorres; page 119 © Marian Weyo
Layout: Jake Flaherty

Contents

CHAPTER 4

Condiments and Sauces **55**

CHAPTER 5

Vinegar Sauces 74

CHAPTER 6

Mayonnaises and Aioli **77**

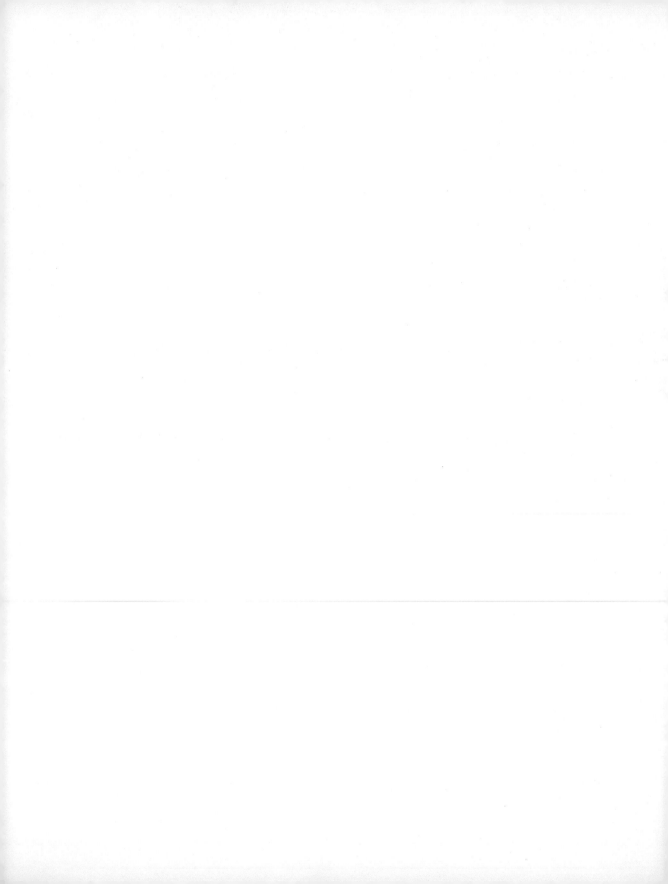

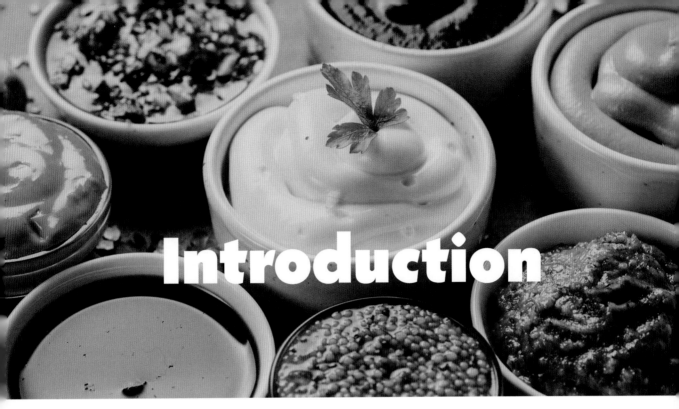

Introduction

As I go into my sixth year of navigating the ketogenic diet, I look back and reflect on the journey thus far. I've seen what the ketogenic diet has done for so many people, and I'm in awe. There are many resources and much more support nowadays than when I first started. When I mention keto, people know what I'm talking about. There are keto specialty shops. Wow! I never thought I'd see that happen.

I think of the many people I've met and befriended because of this diet. I am thankful that it brings together a community of people looking for change, to better themselves, their lives, and the lives of others.

I'm in great health, soon I'll be nine years cancer-free. And that's where I started, my why. I was looking to improve my health somehow when I stumbled upon a Reddit post about the keto diet, and my life has changed since.

I've cooked up a storm, experimenting in the kitchen. I wrote this second cookbook while playing around with recipes and sharing my love of food. The inspiration for this cookbook came when I observed that many mass-produced sauces and dressings have ingredients, such as high-fructose corn syrup, other sugars, and starches, that are counterproductive to the ketogenic diet. It inspired me to go back to basics and learn how to make my own mayonnaise, choosing what goes in it.

For many, the keto diet has similarly entailed moving away from manufactured and processed foods and moving toward more wholesome, home-cooked meals. This is a big step; I've met numerous keto dieters who had never cooked a meal prior to embarking on the keto diet. Inexperience coupled with limited time on a busy schedule can make creating meals with a variety of flavors challenging.

For myself, living in multicultural Vancouver, BC, I've been fortunate to be surrounded by cuisines from varying cultures. This ketogenic condiment, sauces, and rubs cookbook combines my love of food and flavors with the keto diet. Rubs that excite taste buds and sauces that not only add another dimension of flavor but can also aid in fat supplementation. This cookbook will encourage you to try different flavors and experiment by creating some of your own while enjoying the keto diet.

My journey is certainly not over, and I can't wait to see what the future brings. Until then I'll be off in the corner, smoking a brisket and beef ribs with some butter.

If you've been thinking of starting the ketogenic diet, now is the best time. You'll be glad you did and will be looking back months from now thanking yourself.

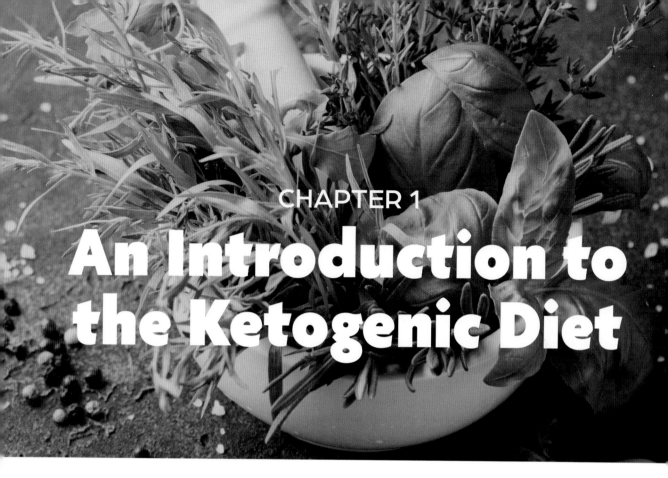

CHAPTER 1
An Introduction to the Ketogenic Diet

The ketogenic diet has gained widespread popularity in the last couple of years. There's been a 1,000% increase in the search for "ketogenic diet" on Google this year, in the U.S. alone, compared to two years ago. Numerous people around the world, including celebrities, athletes, and everyday people alike have tried the diet. While some consider the keto diet another one of those fad diets that come and go, others have found the benefits life changing and have made it their preferred way of eating.

Depending on the individual, benefits of the keto diet may include but are not limited to:

- Better immune system support

- Better sleep quality

- Clearer skin

- Decreased appetite and lack of carb cravings

- Improved digestion

- Improved mental clarity and stability

- Increased energy

- Increased satiety

- Inflammation reduction

- Insulin reduction

- Less bloat
- Lower and more stabilized blood glucose
- Lower blood pressure

- Muscle sparing (Other dieters commonly experience a decrease in muscle mass compared to fat loss. This is not the case with those on the ketogenic diet.)
- Weight loss

Most of all, it doesn't feel like a diet, with plenty of delicious, rich, high-calorie foods to choose from.

It's being used to manage:

- Cancer
- Disease
- Migraines

- Mood disorders
- Polycystic ovarian syndrome
- Seizures

Recent medical studies examining the keto diet show participants not only experience incredible weight loss but also a reduction or complete elimination of ailments and remission of diseases.

People with ailments such as high blood pressure and diseases such as type 2 diabetes, fatty liver disease, metabolic syndrome, hypertension, and heart disease on the keto diet have seen improvements in their conditions. Some oncologists are recommending the keto diet as a tool in conjunction with conventional treatments in cancer management.

In some cases, the research is still in its infancy and more data needs to be obtained. Nonetheless, ongoing research hopes to uncover what this shift in eating can achieve.

What Is the Ketogenic Diet?

At its very essence, the ketogenic diet is a high-fat, moderate-protein, and ultra-low-carbohydrate diet. The calorie intake breakdown is approximately 75% from fat, 20% from protein, and a mere 5% from carbohydrates, which amounts to about 20 to 25 grams of net carbs. This ratio can vary with the individual and their goals.

While there are now a plethora of books and online resources on the ketogenic diet, it is simply eliminating/reducing your carbohydrate intake to about 25 grams of net carbs while increasing fat to the extent where your body switches over from using glucose to fat as a main fuel. These fats are then converted by the liver to ketone bodies, which are acetone, acetoacetate, and beta-hydroxybutyrate, the main ketone that the body uses as fuel. This metabolic fat-burning process is known as ketosis, not to be confused with the serious diabetic medical complication, ketoacidosis.

The ketogenic diet isn't new. Dr. Russell Wilder, a physician at the Mayo Clinic, developed the classic ketogenic diet in the 1920s as a therapy to manage epileptic seizures in children by altering their metabolism, and is still used today.

It can be incredibly confusing and daunting to navigate the plentiful resources and many different methods and ideas about the ketogenic diet that have emerged. Even within the last four to five years, so much has been discovered, and what works best can differ on an individual basis. For example, some dieters have found that 50 grams of net carbohydrates works well for them while others found that 10 grams of total carbohydrates and removing sugar alcohols improves their well-being.

It is a good idea to do some reading beforehand to know what to expect, but not to the point that you're caught up in so much information that it's overwhelming and you never get around to actually starting.

The ketogenic diet is, at its core, quite simple. You can start right away. You don't need pills, shakes, special foods, special tools, or services. Start Simple on page 6 will guide you on how to begin.

While you can pop into ketosis within a mere few days, it can take about four to six weeks to become fat adapted and run efficiently. The body shifts from relying on carbohydrates, after all the glucose in the bloodstream and the glycogen in the liver is metabolized, as a quick fuel source to burning fat. The ketogenic diet isn't one that you can follow Monday to Friday, and then not on the weekends. Doing this would be rough on the body and would not enable it to fully adapt to experience the benefits.

The ketogenic diet is also not a diet that you could "try" for a few days to see if it works. Cheating can be taxing on the body if it results in going in and out of ketosis, as the body prefers the quick-burning carbs as a fuel source. If the ketogenic diet is something that you wish to try, give it an earnest effort for a few months.

Approaches to Keto

There are three different approaches to a ketogenic diet, and they all prescribe to keeping your carb intake between 20 and 25 grams of net carbs.

Strict: Includes tracking macronutrients (also known as macros), which are carbohydrates, fat, and protein, and caloric intake by weighing and measuring all the food you consume, then logging the numbers into a diary or a macro/meal tracker app. For this approach, you'll need to find a macro calculator to determine your personal macros based on your weight, age, height, level of activity, and goals. There are many online keto macro calculators available that are free to use.

Next, you'll need an app to enter your macros and information. Some popular ones include Carb Manager, MyFitnessPal, and Senza, to name a few. Just check your app store to see what would work best for you. In addition to macro tracking, some apps have communities where you can interact with other members and share recipes, tips, tricks, victories, and challenges to support each other.

Lazy: There's no strict calorie or macro tracking involved here, aside from making sure that carb intake stays within 20 to 25 grams. This method consists of choosing foods that are typically low in carbs and maintaining a general idea of how much you can have. This intuitive eating approach is for those who would like the freedom of not counting every single morsel.

Dirty: Includes processed foods and fast foods, as long as they fit within your personal macro allotment.

Over time, you may choose to modify your own approach to keto and do a hybrid or whatever works best for you, whether it's by personal preference or what your body prefers. Focused approaches some dieters have implemented with success are carnivore, vegetarian, vegan, and nondairy, just to name a few. They still keep their total or net carbs restricted to remain in ketosis.

Start Simple

Before you begin, visit your doctor or a medical professional who is familiar with your medical history and the ketogenic diet. Asses if this ultra-low-carb diet is right for you and whether you have any medical conditions that may contradict or interfere with your health while on the diet. You may need to check in with your doctor every so often to monitor your health and progress while on the diet. It's also a good idea to get some baseline bloodwork readings done.

Once you get the green light...what to do next?

Going cold turkey and trying to eliminate all carbs right from the beginning can be quite jarring and frustrating. It can be daunting having to count this and that...and if you go over, you "fail," which can be discouraging. Feeling like you're not doing the diet "perfectly" could cause you to quit. Remember, it's an ongoing learning process.

Start simple with the following steps:

1. ELIMINATE ALL ADDED SUGARS AND PROCESSED FOODS. Added sugars include white refined sugar, brown sugar, corn syrup, agave, maple syrup, and coconut sugar. Skip adding sugar to your coffee and tea. If needed, use a natural alternative sweetener such as stevia or monk fruit.

Processed foods, including salad dressings, marinades, and sauces, contain loads of sugar and starches. There are many names for "sugar" that the body breaks down and uses like glucose. Some common ones are high-fructose corn syrup, corn syrup, dextrose, dextrin, and malto-dextrin. Starches are cornstarch, tapioca, potato, and wheat flour. Not to worry, this cookbook has recipes that will teach you how to make your own sugar-free, keto-friendly, and delicious versions!

Just by implementing this first step of removing added sugars and processed foods, many find that their clothes fit more loosely and they feel better overall.

2. ELIMINATE "DRUNKEN" SOURCES OF CARBOHYDRATES. Sugary drinks such as soda, energy drinks, and juices are so easy to consume and bump up carb intake quickly with just a can. If it helps, transitioning with diet versions of these drinks might prove useful.

Learn about carbohydrate sources and check nutrition labels for carbohydrate content in foods. It's quite the eye-opener to see what foods have hidden carbs in them.

3. ELIMINATE OTHER COMMON CARBOHYDRATES. These include breads, pasta, potatoes, rice, beans, grains, and carbohydrate-heavy fruits and vegetables.

Keto–Friendly Foods

Focusing on what you can't eat can feel incredibly restrictive. There are so many delicious foods that you can eat!

The following lists are by no means exhaustive, but there's enough here to give you a good idea of what you can eat when you're first starting off. Also, keto-friendly foods can differ from individual to individual with sensitivities—you'll slowly learn what works for your body and what doesn't.

PROTEIN: beef, pork, poultry, fish, seafood, eggs, game meats, organ meats.

VEGETABLES: (listed here in order of lowest to highest net carbs: kale, bok choy, lettuce, spinach, asparagus, radishes, zucchini, white mushrooms, cauliflower, eggplant, cucumber, cabbage, broccoli, brussels sprouts, bell peppers.

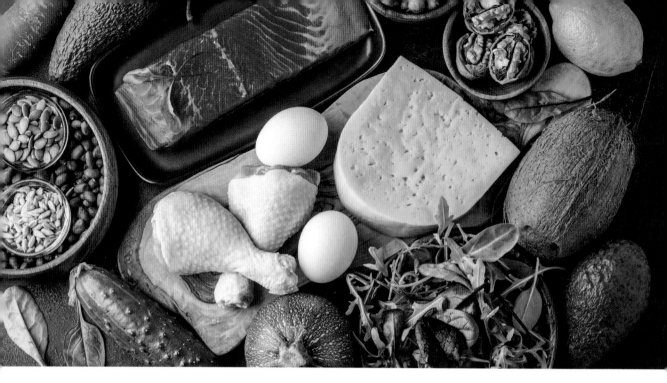

FRUIT: avocado, coconut, and berries in moderation.

DAIRY: full-fat sour cream, hard cheeses, 33% to 35% fat heavy cream.

FATS: avocado, butter, coconut, ghee, lard (rendered pork fat), olives, schmaltz (rendered chicken fat), suet, tallow (rendered beef/mutton fat), some nut oils, MCT (medium-chain triglycerides) oil

NUTS: (good in moderation, listed here in order of lowest to highest net carbs): pili, pecans, Brazil, macadamia, hazelnuts, peanuts, almonds, pine, pistachios, cashews.

OTHER: very dark chocolate, in moderation.

ALCOHOL: (in moderation): low-carb beer, dry red wine, spirits.

Avoiding the Keto Flu

Consuming adequate water, electrolytes, and fat is the key to avoiding the keto flu.

Before the body switches over to using fat as a fuel source, it will use the glucose in the body and any glycogen (stored glucose) reserves in the liver until they are depleted. The glycogen in the liver is stored along with water in a 4 to 1 ratio. Once the glycogen is gone, there is no need to store that water, and it is released. You might experience rapid weight loss in the beginning, it's very likely the result of losing the stored water.

Along with the water, sodium tends to be expelled, which causes an imbalance in electrolytes (sodium, potassium, and magnesium). If you don't stay properly hydrated and your electrolytes aren't supplemented, you may experience symptoms resembling a flu.

Keto flu symptoms can include but are not exclusive to light-headedness, weakness, irritability, headaches, dizziness, muscle cramping, dry mouth, head fogginess, trouble concentrating, insomnia, carb cravings, nausea, and stomach/digestive issues. Depending on the individual, some, none, or all of these might be experienced.

While you can supplement using electrolyte powders, drinks, or pills, which are perfectly acceptable (just check out their ingredient labels for added starch fillers and/or sugars), you can obtain them through food too.

SODIUM: pickles, pickle brine, olives, salt

POTASSIUM: avocados, almonds, broccoli, brussels sprouts, spinach

MAGNESIUM: almonds, spinach, pumpkin seeds

Fat as Fuel

Fat has been demonized for many years. It can be difficult to retrain ourselves to see fat as necessary. Fats, also known as lipids, are needed by the body to build hormones, chemical neurotransmitters, and other essential biomolecules it requires to function properly.

Saturated fats tend to be solid at room temperature. They tend to come from animal-derived products such as butter and lard but also coconut oil and cocoa butter. Saturated fats in particular have had a bad reputation as it was believed that they contributed to heart disease, when in fact they aid in immune and hormone system regulation as well as cell membrane maintenance.

Monounsaturated fats tend to be liquid at room temperature. Oils such as extra-virgin olive oil, avocado oil, and macadamia oil are examples of monounsaturated fats.

Omega-3 and omega-6 are essential polyunsaturated fatty acids. Fatty fish (such as sardines, anchovies, and salmon), grass-fed animals, eggs from grass-fed chickens, chia, and flax are sources of omega-3s. Omega-6s are more plentiful, found in heavily processed vegetable and seed oils as well as the processed foods that include them. There are different thoughts as to the ratio of omega-3 to omega-6 to get. That being said, with omega-6 being quite prevalent in processed foods, it's a good idea to increase your intake of omega-3s.

Fats are even more necessary on the ketogenic diet. While some may have some extra stored body fat that can be used as fuel, the body needs a little help in recognizing that. Supplementing fats in the food we eat will help provide that extra fuel and ensure that fat calorie intake is approximately 75% of total calories consumed. Then by slowly decreasing fat intake, the body will start using fat stores. Fat is incredibly nutrient dense, with 1 gram of fat equal to 9 calories.

In formulating a well-balanced ketogenic diet, choose saturated fats such as butter, ghee, cream, lard, and coconut oil. Include monounsaturated fats such as extra-virgin olive oil and avocado oil. As you increase your intake of fats, particularly animal-derived fats, look for grass-fed varieties because they have higher omega-3 content. Avoid heavily processed vegetable and seed oils such as canola, corn, soy, and sunflower oils. Avoid trans fats.

Remember, on a ketogenic diet, fat is the body's main fuel source. Increasing fat intake doesn't need to be difficult. It can be as simple as cooking with a couple of tablespoons of butter, choosing fattier cuts or grades of protein, reaching for regular ground beef instead of the extra lean, and picking the full-fat cream cheese or sour cream instead of the nonfat or low-fat.

At the table, add a creamy sauce, butter, or olive oil to drizzle on top of your dishes. Top them with nuts, crumbled bacon, or cheese. Have some avocado or olives on the side. Use fatty, creamy sauces to boost fat. This book has several different recipes to cater to different tastes while bringing on the fats. Turn to Mayonnaises and Aioli on page 77 to get started.

Dining Out

Dining out on keto has been getting easier as more restaurants and other food-service establishments have recognized the demand for low-carb foods. Some restaurants have a few keto-friendly offerings, while others have a separate keto menu. If you're fortunate, there may even be a keto restaurant or café in your area. It's refreshing to see.

If there are no keto or low-carb dishes on the menu, mention to the server that you're looking for keto options. They may have some suggestions or alternatives in mind. Sometimes the gluten-free menu might have an option or two that will work.

Generally, choosing a non-breaded protein (beef, lamb, chicken, pork, or fish), plus some low-carb vegetables with butter, or a salad with leafy green vegetables is a good choice. If the protein is sauced, ask if they use any sugars, which includes the likes of honey, maple syrup, and molasses, or starches, such as flour or cornstarch, to thicken. If they do, have them hold the sauce and request a side of butter or olive oil with a little vinegar.

If a dish has a "carby" side, like rice or potato, ask them to hold it or perhaps offer it to a non-keto dining companion.

How to Tell If You're in Ketosis

You can use the following basic ketone body testing methods at home:

- Blood ketone meters monitor the beta-hydroxybutyrate concentration in the blood. The meters are similar to those testing blood glucose, and some can monitor both. A blood ketone concentration reading between 0.5 to 3.0 millimoles per liter (mmol/L) is considered to be in nutritional ketosis.

- Urine test strips monitor the ketone body acetoacetate. It's good when you're first starting out to see if ketone bodies are present. However, these test strips can be inaccurate because the concentration reading changes depending on your hydration level. If there's a positive result, despite the reading, the ketones are flowing.

- Breath meters monitor the ketone body and acetone concentration in your breath. Ketone breath meters are an alternative for those looking for a way to test for ketones without blood or urine.

If you are experiencing some or all of these signs, this can also indicate that you are in ketosis. Again, it can differ between individuals.

- Mental clarity

- Decrease in appetite

- Increase in energy

- Decrease in sleep duration

- Decrease or lack of carb cravings

- Dry mouth

- Acetone-smelling breath and/or urine

- Quick weight loss, initially from the loss of stored water (increased urination frequency can also contribute)

- Experiencing some keto flu symptoms

As your body adapts, you will become familiar with what you are able to eat. You may want to expand your menu options to include no- or low-carb versions of carb-laden foods.

Tracking Your Progress on the Ketogenic Diet

There's nothing more motivating than seeing results! Tracking your progress on the ketogenic diet is more than just watching the scale move. Body weight naturally fluctuates throughout the day so it's good to monitor your progress in multiple ways.

WEIGHT: Weigh yourself during the same time each day. It's best to do within a few hours of waking.

BODY MEASUREMENTS: Take your starting measurements. You'll need a tape measure, somewhere to jot down your measurements, such as a notebook or an app, and a friend to help measure those hard-to-reach places. Look online for how to take body measurements so you'll be able to take them correctly and consistently. Areas you might want to measure are your neck, chest, bust, biceps, wrist, waist, hips, and thighs. You'll want to take measurements weekly or twice a month to monitor progress.

BODY FAT PERCENTAGE: There are several methods to figure out body fat percentage. One of the best ways is via a DEXA scan, a low-energy x-ray scan used to determine bone density and to identify body composition where you can also see where the fat resides. The con of getting a DEXA scan is that they can be quite pricey, and it can be challenging to find a nearby facility that's able to do one.

Smarter body weight scales on the market are able to estimate body fat percentage via bioelectrical impedance, where a weak electrical current is sent through the body and the voltage reading is converted to body fat percentage based on your height and total weight. These readings can be tracked via an app associated with the scale. Skinfold measurements have been used to estimate body fat percentage for years. By pinching the skin with the aid of skinfold calipers to measure underlying fat in different locations around the body, such as the triceps, abdomen, and thigh, you can estimate body fat percentage. This method can be tricky as it's best to have someone take the measurements on you for best results. The more measurements taken around the body, the better the body fat estimate. Though this method is simple and somewhat quick, it needs some experience to achieve accurate results.

While you can get caught up in accuracy, it's good to get a basic idea and just watch where the trend line goes!

BLOOD TESTS: If you have certain medical concerns, simple blood tests such as blood glucose readings, A1C, LDL, total cholesterol, triglycerides, etc., will provide you with a starting baseline. Have those initial readings/tests done before you start with the advice and supervision of a medical professional. Then have those tests done again after a predetermined time period on the ketogenic diet, and discuss the results with your medical professional.

PICTURES: Take starting pictures. Start with the front of your body, then continue with the right side, back, and left side. You may need to enlist the help of a friend to take back photos or use a mirror or a camera with a tripod and timer. Next, take a picture of your face. Keep in mind that these photos are for your eyes only! There's a good chance that you'll immediately want to delete these starting pictures, but don't! Store them away. Then every week, take progress photos and compare them with your starting point. Trust me, you'll be glad you did. You'll come to notice subtle changes as time goes by.

GOAL CLOTHES: Perhaps having a piece or two of goal clothing works for you. When you don't think you're seeing progress, try on that goal dress or pair of jeans. You just may surprise yourself. It's been observed that what may look like a stall might not be one. If the numbers on the scale look like they haven't moved in a couple of weeks but your clothes are fitting much more loosely, that's a great motivator to keep going!

NAVIGATING A STALL

A stall is when you haven't seen progress in any metric (i.e., weight loss, body measurement loss, etc.) for more than 3 to 4 weeks. Here are some ways to troubleshoot the stall:

If you're not keeping a food diary, keep track of what and how much you're eating for a few days. That will give you a snapshot to look at. Here are a few ideas and places to start:

- Hydration: Stay hydrated, drink 8 to 10 glasses of water a day. The body needs water to function, and one of those functions is fat breakdown.

- Not eating enough: The body needs fuel to function. If you're not getting enough nutrients to fuel your systems, metabolism slows down and you are not going to lose weight. It's a survival instinct.

- Not in ketosis anymore: How much and how often do you "cheat"? Sneaking a bite of a non-keto cookie, a slice of pizza, or a handful of chips now and then can add up over the course of a day.

- "Carb creep" is quite common if you're not tracking. It can happen especially with eyeballing portion sizes. You may think that it's only one serving when it's three. Or perhaps, it's eating too many sugar alcohols or the wrong sugar alcohols for your body. Though a particular food may be considered a keto treat, having one might be enough for you. Too many and that can pop you out of ketosis. There also might be hidden carbs in the foods you're ingesting.

Celebrate Your Progress

What should you do if the keto diet is working really well for you and you're running out of clothes that fit? Check out thrift stores! There was a time when I couldn't even button up a pair of jeans at the beginning of a month, and by month's end, those jeans were so big that I needed a belt to keep them on my waist.

Don't compare your results with those of other people. Everyone is different and will see progress differently too. You can lose motivation comparing yourself to someone who started their keto journey earlier than you and who's seeing significant changes when you've only just begun.

To keep things fresh or to keep yourself motivated, you might want to set up non-food rewards when you reach specific milestones. An example would be a manicure/pedicure at 10 pounds lost or a special excursion at 50 pounds lost. What and which ones you want to celebrate are entirely up to you.

Don't give up! Celebrate your progress along the way no matter how small.

Part of success is feeding yourself appropriately and not feeling deprived. Try to keep a normal routine and substitute foods that are keto-friendly. In some cases, you'll need to find or simply make your own keto-friendly version. Eating unprocessed food is a start. Over time you'll want to mix things up a bit and try different ideas for variety. Changing up your seasonings and sauces can keep your palate interested and keep you from getting bored. It can be a challenge to find keto-friendly store-bought spice mixes and sauces—the next time you're grocery shopping, take a look at the ingredients label and nutrition panel. This cookbook is here to help!

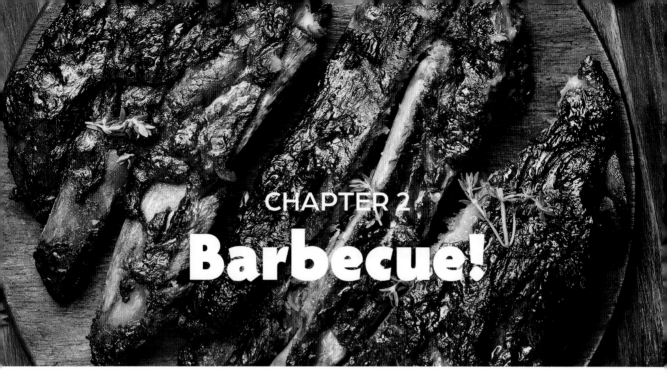

CHAPTER 2

Barbecue!

Whether you're talking about the cooking style or the outdoor gathering of friends around food, barbecue feels like the celebration of summer! There's nothing like food cooked over a flame, and everyone enjoys good barbecue.

I'd imagine that barbecue has been around as long as the discovery of fire. Across the years and throughout many cultures, traditional barbecue consists of cooking outdoors over a grill or in a pit, with wood or coals.

There are different thoughts on barbecue, with some folks who are passionate and take their barbecue very personally and seriously. As they should! Cooking a brisket low and slow for 12 to 14 hours with all the care and attention is a labor of love.

Whether you decide to go low and slow for hours over a wood-burning smoker or hit the high heat on a grill, there are rubs, marinades, sauces, and condiments that not only add flavor but also bring out the best in your ingredients.

Though the search is getting easier than it was when I first started over four years ago, finding keto-friendly sauces and seasonings can feel like looking for a needle in a haystack. Skimming over an ingredient label from a store-bought barbecue sauce, you'll find high-fructose corn syrup as the first ingredient. (Ingredients are listed on the label in order of most to least abundant.) Looking at the rest of the ingredients on the label, there's modified cornstarch (a thickener), corn syrup, molasses, and sugar among the seasonings and recognizable flavors. Looking at the nutrition panel, there are 18 grams of carbs per 2-tablespoon serving, of which 16 grams comes from sugar.

If you're tracking carbohydrate intake and trying to stick to 20 grams of net carbs, 2 tablespoons of this sauce alone is 90% of that.

Making your own sauces from scratch is satisfying and fun, plus you can exercise some creativity in the kitchen.

Components of Sauces

Anatomy of sauce: It's all about balance. Balance of flavor, balance between the sauce and the food you're serving it with, and what you like.

The ingredients listed here will give you an idea of what to use in your sauces for salty, sour, sweet, bitter, umami, and heat elements. Hopefully, over time, you'll start to experiment and get creative with your sauce making.

Keep in mind, some ingredients add more than one element, which builds layers of flavor. Most especially, hold back before adding salt, especially if you are using ingredients that are naturally salty too. Taste the sauce first, then assess if more salt is needed.

If you've never tried some of these ingredients, give them a try. You might find your next favorite ingredient.

Salty

ANCHOVIES/ANCHOVY PASTE: A small oily fish high in omega-3 fatty acids that is packed with flavor. The canned variety is packed in salt but also has an umami punch. It can be fishy and a little overwhelming. Use smaller amounts to start to bring out the best of your ingredients, then adjust to your preference.

COCONUT AMINOS: Made by the fermentation of salted sap from coconut blossoms, this savory sauce is comparable to soy sauce, without the soy.

FISH SAUCE: Fermenting salted fish for a few years is the secret of what makes this sauce incredibly savory. Though it imparts a saltiness, it's used more often for its umami characteristics.

LIQUID AMINOS/GLUTEN-FREE TAMARI: Both are made from soybeans (without wheat, unlike soy sauce) and are another substitute for soy sauce. Note: some tamaris have some wheat.

SEA SALT/HIMALAYAN SALT: Both salts contain naturally occurring, beneficial trace minerals and no added fillers or additives, unlike table salt.

SHRIMP PASTE: Made by fermenting small shrimp and occasionally small fish with salt for a few weeks, a fermentation process that concentrates its natural umami characteristics. Very little goes a long, long way to enhance flavor.

Sour

APPLE CIDER VINEGAR: One would think that this would contain quite a few carbs being from apples, but it's the contrary. This vinegar is made from fermented apple juice where bacteria and yeast convert the sugars to acetic acid. The complex flavors from the fermentation process add a wonderful umami layer of flavor along with the sourness.

BALSAMIC VINEGAR: Made from white grapes, including seeds, juice, stems, and skins, and fermented, this is jam-packed with incredible flavor that itself has elements of sour, sweet, and umami. But be aware that it has a higher carbohydrate content than other vinegars, with 2.7 grams carbs per tablespoon. Not to worry, it's rich in flavor and a little goes a long way.

CITRIC ACID: Not to be mistaken for ascorbic acid (vitamin C), though both are primarily obtained from citrus fruit. You may already be familiar with citric acid as it's used as a natural food preservative and to reduce fruit browning. Good for adding a level of tanginess/tartness that gets you to pucker up.

LEMON/LIMES: Citrus fruits brighten sauces with their acidity without adding too many carbs. Use the zest to concentrate those flavors without adding carbs.

PICKLE BRINE: Its uses are often underestimated. Don't toss it out when all the pickles are gone. It's great to help with electrolyte balance while adding a salty, spicy acidity.

RICE VINEGAR: Made by the fermentation of rice, rice vinegar adds a few elements. A sourness along with a little sweetness and some umami characteristics too.

WHITE VINEGAR: Straight, clean, uncomplicated acidity, adding a crisp sourness without carbs. It's made by fermenting alcohol or sugar by bacteria. Acetic acid diluted down to 5%.

Sweet

BERRIES: Berries are low in carbs and add a natural sweetness.

SWEETENERS: It can be challenging to look for a keto-friendly sweet alternative for balance that doesn't impart a negative effect and/or flavor. See Sweeteners on page 21 to help you choose those that not only work but also are right for you.

Bitter

Bitter isn't usually a flavor profile that's sought out, but it can help to balance flavor.

HERBS: Herbs add aromatic flavors that can be bitter. Thyme, for example, can be bitter, especially when used in larger amounts.

MUSTARD POWDER: While the bitterness is subdued in prepared mustards, it's strong in powdered mustard.

Umami

What exactly is umami? Often coined as the fifth taste or flavor profile, umami is detected by the tongue, adding to the usual bitter, salty, sweet, and sour profiles. This fifth flavor profile has a savoriness that has been described as "meaty." Umami has been associated with glutamates, which are naturally occurring, broken-down proteins in some foods, resulting in amino acid building blocks. One in particular is glutamic acid. The sodium salt form of glutamic acid is notoriously known as monosodium glutamate (MSG). MSG is somewhat controversial in that it has been thought to cause certain reactions in individuals, such as headaches, but overall has been considered safe by the FDA.

These amino acids impart a savoriness like no other. Umami is found in fish, shellfish, tomatoes, soy, aged cheeses, and fermented foods. Fermenting a food with a natural umami component will concentrate the umami flavors. Shrimp paste is a good example. It's incredibly "fragrant" to say the least. The flavor is fantastic but as I mentioned before, use it very sparingly to create that savoriness.

ANCHOVIES/ANCHOVY PASTE: see Salty (page 16)

FISH SAUCE: see Salty (page 16)

LIQUID AMINOS: see Salty (page 16)

MUSHROOM POWDER: Mushrooms have naturally occurring glutamates (shiitake mushrooms tend to have higher content than most mushrooms), and dehydrating them concentrates their umami profile. Powdered mushrooms provide a convenient method to add that umami punch. A little goes a long way.

OLIVES: Typically, olives are brined or fermented.

PARMESAN CHEESE: Hardened cheeses are aged. Their moisture content is low, so they tend to have a higher umami profile.

SHRIMP PASTE: see Salty (page 16)

TOMATOES/SUNDRIED TOMATOES: Tomatoes naturally contain glutamic acid. Drying them with the sun, food dehydrator, or low oven concentrates the glutamates. Dry sundried tomatoes need to be hydrated with some water before using. Those packed in olive oil are ready to use.

WORCESTERSHIRE SAUCE: Fermented anchovies are the main ingredient in this sauce.

Heat

BLACK PEPPERCORNS: Readily available, these are not as hot as capsaicin–containing chili peppers, but piperine gives them that spicy heat. Crack them in a pepper or spice grinder.

CHILI PASTES: Simply made from ground chilies, they may contain other ingredients like vinegar or other seasonings. Sambal oelek is a popular Indonesian chili paste that's easy to use. Just grab a spoon and scoop it in.

CHILI POWDER: A combination of cayenne, chipotle, habanero, serrano, and Scotch bonnet.

CHINESE PEPPERCORNS: While not hot, these peppercorns have the unique characteristic of causing a slight tingly/numbing sensation on the lips and tongue to mimic the sensation of spiciness.

FRESH CHILIES: Bring on the heat! Chilies contain capsaicin, which stimulates the tongue to perceive that heat. To reduce the level of heat in your recipe, you can choose to remove the seeds and ribs (the white bits that hold the seeds) as the capsaicin tends to be found in higher concentration in these parts.

HORSERADISH ROOT/WASABI RHIZOME: Horseradish and wasabi come from the same plant family (Brassicaceae) and stimulate the olfactory senses whereas capsaicin in chilies stimulate the tongue.

HOT SAUCES: I've seen the variety of hot sauces in the marketplace go up exponentially in the last 10 years, and it's wonderful to see more than just the usual tabasco chili pepper hot sauce to choose from. Just check the ingredients label for sugar or other, sugar–like sweeteners. While 2 teaspoons might be all you need for the entire recipe, the sugar impact might be minimal for some or greater for others. Just go with what works for you.

MUSTARD: Mustard comes from the same family as horseradish and wasabi and therefore stimulates the senses in the same way. Usually, the milder white mustard seeds are used to make the commonly known prepared mustard, while brown and black mustard seeds have a hotter kick.

PICKLED CHILIES: The bonus with pickled chilies is that the spicy brine can be used too!

Fats

AVOCADO OIL: Avocados are naturally high in fat, monounsaturated fat in particular. So, it comes as no surprise that it's somewhat easy to press avocados to extract the oil. Avocado oil is good general all-purpose oil with a nice, high smoke point and a somewhat neutral flavor.

BUTTER/GHEE: There's nothing like the rich flavor of butter, with or without salt. Add another dimension and use browned butter for a nuttier take. Ghee is clarified butter with the milk solids removed. It keeps a little longer and has a higher smoke point than butter.

COCONUT OIL: Contains healthy saturated fats that are especially beneficial to ketosis. Though it may impart a flavor and it becomes solid at lower temperatures.

CREAM: The fattiest cream coming in at 33% to 35% milk fat, it's usually known as heavy cream or whipping cream. Check the ingredient list as it may contain emulsifiers and/or starches that help it to retain its shape when whipped.

LARD: Rendered pork fat. It may not be easy to find where you live but it's easy to render yourself. Just place some pork fat from the butcher in a slower cooker set to low. Once liquid, strain out any bits and store it covered in the fridge for two to three months or in the freezer for a couple of years. If you can get leaf lard, you've hit the jackpot. It is rendered fat from around the kidneys. There's no flavor, and it consists of a light color and texture that's spreadable.

MCT OIL: Medium chain triglycerides usually consist of C6, C8, C10, and C12 triglycerides refined from coconuts that the body uses readily when in ketosis. It has no flavor, which makes it perfect to use. Keep in mind that it can be a little pricey compared to other oils. If you're new to using MCT oil, introduce it slowly as it has been known to cause tummy aches or digestive upset, particularly the varieties containing C6 triglycerides. If you find that you're sensitive to regular MCT oil, look into those that only contain C8 or a combination of C8 and C10 triglycerides.

OLIVE OIL: Extra-virgin olive oil comes from the first press of olives and tends to be the most flavorful and expensive. It's not recommended for cooking over other oils that are less expensive, more neutral in flavor, and have a higher smoke point. It's best in dressings where there's no cooking involved and the flavor comes through best.

TALLOW: Usually made by rendering animal fat (except pork, which is called lard). This is a nice saturated fat made similarly to lard by slow melting/cooking the fat in a slow cooker over several hours and straining out the solid bits. Tallow has a high smoke point and tends to be solid at room temperature.

Thickeners

GUAR GUM: Extracted from guar beans, this is a common thickener. Very little is needed per use (¼ teaspoon per quart or liter of liquid).

XANTHAN GUM: Usually derived from the fermentation of glucose and sucrose, it's used as a thickener and emulsifier. Use in very small amounts (¼ teaspoon of xanthan gum for every 2 cups of liquid), and sprinkle it in while mixing to incorporate it evenly and prevent clumping.

SHORT CUT!

Using commercially available sauces as a base to build on can be a great idea. There's more variety in the marketplace for the health conscious. Just have a look at that ingredient label and nutritional panel to see if the sauce works for you.

If you're strict and need to eliminate all bulk-made commercial sources then don't use it. Also, if you're sensitive to some or any of these then they're definitely not an option. If you're not, it may be something you wish to use but when added to other sources of carbs, the total of your intake might be just enough to keep you out of the ketosis metabolic state.

Not to worry, starting on page 31, you can learn to make rubs, marinades, and sauces from scratch using a range of base ingredients.

Sweeteners

Switching over to the ketogenic diet can be difficult initially due to the prevalence of the sugars found in our day-to-day diets. We've gotten used to the taste of sweet things, and eliminating them can take some getting used to. Rather than forgo it all, it can help to use a sweetener, whether artificial or natural, that has minimal or no impact on blood sugar to help you through those tough moments. Sugar alcohol is one such option because of its structure. Some sugar alcohols are naturally occurring and are extracted and isolated. Some people are sensitive and have had digestive issues. In some cases, its merely a matter of getting used to it and in other cases, the body just doesn't agree with it.

ALLULOSE: A rare natural sweetener found in small amounts in dried fruits such as raisins and figs. It's relatively new to the marketplace and has not been found to affect blood sugar levels. It replaces sugar 1:1.

ERYTHRITOL: A natural sweetener that's been found in small amounts in fruit; also a by-product of the fermentation of glucose by yeast. It's 70% sweeter than sugar, has no aftertaste, and has a cooling effect. It doesn't affect blood glucose levels.

SUCRALOSE: A chemically manufactured sweetener that's about 1,000 times sweeter than sugar. It's not retained by the body so it's considered noncaloric. Sucralose is combined with a filler for the powdered form, which does have some carbs. The liquid version does not.

STEVIA: A natural sweetener from the stevia plant that's 150 times sweeter than sugar. It has a very low impact on blood sugar. Though it has a distinctive aftertaste, this might not be noticed as much in a sauce or when used with another sweetener.

MONK FRUIT: Named after the fruit it's found in, monk fruit is 200 times sweeter than sugar. Monk fruit doesn't affect blood glucose levels. It has a very light, almost fruity aftertaste.

XYLITOL: A natural sweetener found in small amounts in some fruits. It doesn't spike blood sugar and is a 7 on the glycemic index scale. The glycemic index is a scale from 0 to 100 where foods are assigned a number that illustrates the rise in blood glucose levels two hours after consumption. Sugar is given the value of 100. To dogs, it is very dangerous and can be lethal.

SWEETENERS IN SAUCES

Sweeteners used alone for cooking and baking may have an aftertaste or sensation. But using them with another sweetener can mask the aftertaste.

I prefer to use Swerve for sauce making. It's primarily erythritol and prebiotic oligosaccharides. It replaces sugar 1 to 1 and has no impact on blood sugar. Swerve makes a brown "sugar" version that is rich in flavor and works quite well as a substitute for brown sugar and honey. There are other brown sugar substitutes and sugar-free syrups in the marketplace if Swerve doesn't work for you. Some other examples of brown sugar substitutes are Sukrin Gold and Lakanto Golden. Some golden syrup substitutes are Lakanto Maple-Flavored Syrup, Good Dee's Sugar Free Syrup, Walden Farms, and ChocZero.

Herbs and Spices

Herbs and spices come from edible plants that add a flavor dimension to cooking by harmonizing with other ingredients. Due to their aromatic nature, even a little can deliver a ton of zest. The majority of sauces, marinades, and rubs use some herb and/or spice. Once you get accustomed to using them, you'll want to try more.

Herbs are mostly the leaves and, sometimes, stems of the plant. Spices are everything else: the roots, seeds, and bark of the plant.

Fresh vs. Dried

Fresh is always nicer, though one drawback is availability. Even with local greenhouses growing them all year round, fresh herbs are scooped up quickly. Another challenge is quality. With the high demand on local growers, many grocery stores bring them in from elsewhere and by the time they reach your cart, they may not be at their best for very long. If you have the desire, you can grow fresh herbs at home too.

Having a collection of dried herbs and spices is certainly convenient. Keep in mind that dried herbs are more concentrated since the process of drying them removes water, making them more compact. A general rule to remember is that dried herbs are three times more concentrated than fresh, so 1 teaspoon dried = 1 tablespoon fresh (since a tablespoon measure is equivalent to 3 teaspoons).

1 teaspoon dried herbs = 1 tablespoon fresh herbs

Both herbs and spices contain fragrant aromatics that bring scent and flavor. These aromatics are usually best when they're fresh, but in some cases, such as when they're not in season or if they don't grow where you live, fresh isn't ideal or convenient, especially when you're putting together proteins that need to go in the smoker at 5:30 a.m.

For dried herbs and spices, check through your pantry. Do you still have those original herbs and spices in the spice rack gift you received at your housewarming eons ago? Do they look faded? Are they clumped up? The more important question is: are they still good?

Some manufacturers are adding "best before" dates to their bottles but you should also check the spices for their potency as it can change with storage.

According to the FoodKeeper app by the USDA, the shelf life of whole spices is three to four years, and the shelf life of ground spices is two to three years.

Old herbs and spices don't normally go bad unless there's moisture present. They become less potent, as they lose their aromatic essence over time.

Visual indications include color or clumping. Green herbs look faded, red spices look brown. If they're cakey and clumping, it indicates that moisture is present. Sometimes, moist herbs get moldy. It's best to discard those.

To check its effectiveness, take a liberal pinch of the herb or spice then place it in the palm of your hand. Rub it a little to activate any oils present, and then smell it.

If the scent is bright and vibrant, you're good to go. If it smells a little muted and dull, it's faded but you can still use it if you're stuck. Just use more to bring out the flavor, and be aware that using more may change the texture of your sauces or change the spice ratio in rubs, and you may need to adjust. If there's no smell, it's completely stale. It won't add anything, so discard.

Purchasing Herbs and Spices

Start your spice collection with the following if you don't have any:

- Black peppercorns and black pepper
- Chili powder (not seasoning, which is a blend)
- Chili flakes
- Garlic
- Ginger
- Onion
- Oregano
- Paprika
- Thyme

The little glass bottles in the grocery store can be really expensive and may seem like an investment when you don't have anything and are just starting out. Here are a few tips to get quality herbs and spices without breaking the bank.

- Ethnic stores tend to have larger bags for great prices.
- Online stores often package up their spices on demand to retain freshness. They tend to have a larger variety and offer specialty items. For example, they will list the spice and the location where it was grown, lending to subtle differences in their flavor.
- Bargain stores are inexpensive, but look for quality. Check the "best before" date on the bottle if there is one.
- Check the quality: Are they all stems? The stems can be woody and have limited flavor.
- Check the container: They're inexpensive when sold in bags instead of containers. Will you need to transfer them later? If you won't be using it all within a couple of weeks, transfer the remainder into an airtight container.
- Bulk: Sure, the big-box store has a big shaker bottle for a fabulous price. Will you use it fast enough before it reaches its best before date? Fantastic, for longer-storage spices like black peppercorns. For a home cook, usually a few ounces will suffice. Pick up larger amounts of your most-used spices as we tend to gravitate toward our favorites.
- Whole spices (e.g., seeds, bark, etc.) last a little longer when they're kept whole. This includes spices such as nutmeg, coriander seed, fennel seed, cloves, and peppercorns.

Storing Herbs and Spices

When storing herbs and spices, keep them away from light, heat, and moisture. Do not place them on top of the stove or by the sink, dishwasher, or fridge. If the product does not have a manufacturer's "best before" date, mark the spice with the date your purchased it or, if you harvested the herb yourself, the date you bottled it.

GLASS: Glass jars with a tight lid to keep out air and moisture for a longer term for those spices you don't use as often are optimal. Small canning jars work great.

METAL: This is a good option as long as it isn't a salt blend, which can corrode the metal.

PLASTIC: Plastic containers are porous and the aromatics can dissipate, making them go stale more quickly. Avoid storing herbs and spices in plastic bags. Plastic bags are more porous than hard plastic containers, and when stored next to other herbs in bags, they all start to smell the same.

Using Herbs and Spices

1. Toast them over dry heat to bring out oils.

2. Don't shake spices directly over a steaming pot. The spices absorb the hot steam, which reduces their potency and shelf life quicker. It can cause clumping too. Perhaps sprinkle some into your hand to warm them up, then sprinkle them in.

3. Use a spice mill or spice grinder or a mortar and pestle to break down whole spices.

Growing Herbs

One easy luxury is growing herbs yourself. Benefits: It's fresh and inexpensive. Just clip what you need and know that you're getting organic quality.

There's nothing like having a constant supply of fresh basil over the summer to make fresh pesto. Spoil yourself over those summer months. You don't need an elaborate garden. If you're in a small space, window boxes or plant pots on a small patio work really well. You can find kits for growing herbs indoors at home and can even monitor your plants via Bluetooth and an app.

To start, plant seeds or pick up seedlings in the spring from the local nursery. Perennial herbs such as chives, thyme, sage, and rosemary don't need to be planted every year depending on where you live. They keep coming back every year making it really easy to have fresh herbs every summer with minimal effort.

Use what you need and with an abundance, preserve for the rest of the year.

Storing Herbs

Don't let fresh herbs go bad in their plastic packaging from the store. Here are some tips for storing herbs:

FREEZING: Chop and place premeasured portions in an ice cube tray then fill with water or melted butter. Hardy herbs like basil, parsley, thyme, and rosemary work really well with this method.

Make a few compound butter mixes and freeze them. Ginger also keeps in the freezer; grate as needed.

DRYING: Spread the herbs on a parchment paper–covered cookie sheet in a low-temperature (about 200°F) oven for two to three hours or until dry.

DEHYDRATING: Thyme, rosemary, sage, parsley, cilantro, and chives dry well in a food dehydrator. Basil is tricky and tends to go black before it dries. After drying, store the herbs in a glass jar with a tight-fitting lid labeled with the date.

HOW TO MEASURE FRESH HERBS

Do you pack fresh leafy herbs such as parsley and basil into measuring cups when measuring?

For ease, lightly chop leafy herbs, gently pack, and fill the measuring cup to the top. Fresh herbs have a little bit of give and, usually, a little less or a little more won't make that much of a difference.

Helpful Kitchen Tools

Having the best tools for the job makes sauce preparation so much easier and faster. Here's a list of a few kitchen tools that I use often.

BLENDER: A mid-range, 500-watt blender will blend sauces smooth and emulsify mayonnaise.

CHEESECLOTH: Versatile and inexpensive, it's good for straining out large spices, squeezing out water from grated cucumber, and creating a breathable cover with an elastic band. Always keep some on hand. They're also great to use as an impromptu herb and spice bag (similar to a tea bag) to easily remove infusing herbs and spices.

CITRUS REAMER: This is one of those tools that you don't think you need until you receive one as a gift. Sure, you can absolutely use a fork to juice a lemon but a citrus reamer extracts the juice so much more quickly and efficiently, with little effort.

CONTAINERS: When making your own sauces, it's nice to have containers to hold them. Canning jars are incredibly versatile, with different sizes (from 2 ounces to 64 ounces) and shapes. Some styles have liquid measurements etched on them too. The jars are built to withstand cold and hot temperatures. They've been around for a long time and can be found at garage sales for pennies. For standard regular and wide-mouth sizes, you can find a variety of lids, including lids with spouts for sauces and condiments, and lids with holes for shaking out seasonings.

DIGITAL KITCHEN SCALE: For exact measuring and consistency. Helpful when measuring out portion sizes. Many have an 11-pound (5-kilogram) capacity and weigh 0.05-ounce (1-gram) increments. There are smaller scales that measure down to 0.01 grams, which is helpful when measuring dry spices too light to register on the larger scale.

DIGITAL KITCHEN THERMOMETER: Instantly check the internal temperature of proteins to make sure they are safe to consume.

FLEXIBLE CHOPPING BOARD: After fine-chopping cups of herbs like the parsley needed for chimichurri, this board makes herb transfer effortless.

FOOD PROCESSOR: Small food processors (about 2-cup size) are quite inexpensive and relatively low in power compared to their larger counterparts. While they're not powerful enough to make nut butter or to shred a cabbage, they're incredibly handy and simple to use when making a cup of mayonnaise or pesto, especially when you don't want to haul out the larger appliance. They are easier to wash too.

GARLIC PRESS: Fairly easy to use, place a garlic clove in the hopper and squeeze. What's even easier is that most models don't require you to peel the garlic clove. This can be a lifesaver when you need to crush a few cloves and want to keep your hands from smelling like garlic.

VINYL OR NITRILE GLOVES: Cutting up chilies without gloves can be quite the experience, especially when you have dry hands. Gloves will protect your hands when handling chilies, and they're nice to have on when handling raw meats.

IMMERSION/STICK BLENDER: Safely break down and blend sauces right in the pot on the stove. No need to worry about the dangers of transferring a hot mixture and blending it.

MICROPLANE FINE GRATER: Great for citrus zesting and grating fresh ginger, whole spices, and garlic. The small size creates fluffy zest and fine spice sizes that seem to melt into sauces. No big chunks.

MORTAR AND PESTLE: Tired of chasing peppercorns or coriander seeds around the kitchen with a mallet or a knife? A mortar and pestle just may provide the solution you're looking for.

Fantastic for cracking and pulverizing seeds and spices with ease. Especially a pestle with a little weight to it. Also therapeutic in smashing avocados silky smooth. Easy to clean.

MEASURING SPOONS: Have a couple of sets handy, one for dry ingredients and another for wet ingredients. To use measuring spoons with dry ingredients, fill the spoon and level it off with a butter knife. It can be tricky with dried herbs such as whole rosemary, but it's helpful when using powdered garlic.

KNIFE: In many cases, a chef's or Santoku knife will get the job done. Never underestimate the value, versatility, and ease of a good knife. Keep it sharp and honed.

SAUCE MOP: When the capacity of a basting brush is not enough and you don't want to keep the barbecue lid open for long and lose that precious heat, this tool is helpful to quickly slather moisture to keep those large proteins from drying out during a long and slow cook.

SAUCE SQUEEZE BOTTLES: Keep those condiments like ketchup, mayonnaise, and mustard tidy in easy-to-squeeze bottles.

SHAKER CONTAINER: Disperse rubs evenly and cleanly.

SILICONE OR NATURAL BRISTLE BASTING BRUSH: Silicone can withstand high temperatures and can handle the heat of the grill and the dishwasher.

SPATULA (SMALL): They're great for getting the last bits of mayonnaise out of measuring cups and small dishes with tight edges, like ramekins.

SPRAY BOTTLE: Made of food-safe plastic, use this for spraying moisture on your proteins to prevent them from drying out, especially when smoking for long periods of time.

STRAINER (SMALL): A small metal mesh strainer is helpful to strain out a small amount of solid, like spices and chili flakes.

WET AND DRY MEASURING CUPS: There's a difference between wet and dry measuring cups. Using a dry measuring cup can be tricky measuring liquids and transferring them without spilling. A wet measuring cup is usually glass or plastic with several markings on the side and a pour spout. To use a dry measuring cup, fill it up and level it off with a butter knife. While not essential for cooking, it is for baking.

WHISK: Keep a medium and small whisk, for small amounts, like a cup. They fit in smaller bowls and containers to mix those sauces thoroughly.

Nutritional Information

With most of the recipes, I've included nutritional information as a guide only. It should give you an idea of what to expect.

For example, this is the nutritional information for pesto aioli:

Nutrition Per Serving: Calories: 106 | Net Carbohydrates: 0.8g | Fat: 11g | Protein: 0.9g | Total Carbohydrates: 1g | Fiber: 0.2g

Macros will differ depending on the ingredients you use. For example, you may decide to use a commercially available sugar–free ketchup, or the type and size of produce you use could vary from the recipe. If you do track macros, I suggest calculating them for the ingredients that you use for increased accuracy.

Net carbohydrates were calculated by subtracting the fiber value from carbohydrates (total carbs, which doesn't include erythritol (see Use of Erythritol/Swerve on page 30).

If you're not sure where to find nutritional information for non–packaged ingredients, I suggest using FoodData Central, the USDA's database, which can be found at https://fdc.nal.usda.gov. The website has information on some packaged ingredients too.

A few factors to keep in mind regarding nutritional information and portion sizes:

RUBS: Rubs remain on the surface and the portion size will vary as to how much you'll actually eat as well as how much rub was used (i.e., lightly sprinkled or caked on). For example, think of the amount of rub on the surface of a chicken breast compared to a couple of slices of brisket.

MARINADES: The majority of the marinade is discarded before cooking. Very little marinade is actually left on the surface after cooking.

SAUCES: When cooking with sauces, how much of the sauce is left on the food surface after cooking? Perhaps a teaspoon or two?

If you're adding the sauce at on at the table, I've estimated a 1– to 2–tablespoon portion size. For hot sauces and mustards, since those are usually used in smaller amounts (unless you're a hot sauce fiend) compared to creamier sauces, I've used 1 to 2 teaspoons as the portion size in calculating macros.

Use of Erythritol/Swerve

For the majority of these recipes, I use Swerve, which is erythritol combined with a filler known as prebiotic oligosaccharides. For many people, erythritol works well and isn't retained by the body. Because of this, I don't include it in the carb count at all. If you're counting total carbs, you'll want to include it in your calculations.

If you use a different sweetener that works better for you and has carbs associated with it, such as xylitol, you may need to account for it in the carb macronutrient count if it impacts you. Remember, to dogs, xylitol is dangerous and can be lethal. Please visit the Sweeteners section on page 21.

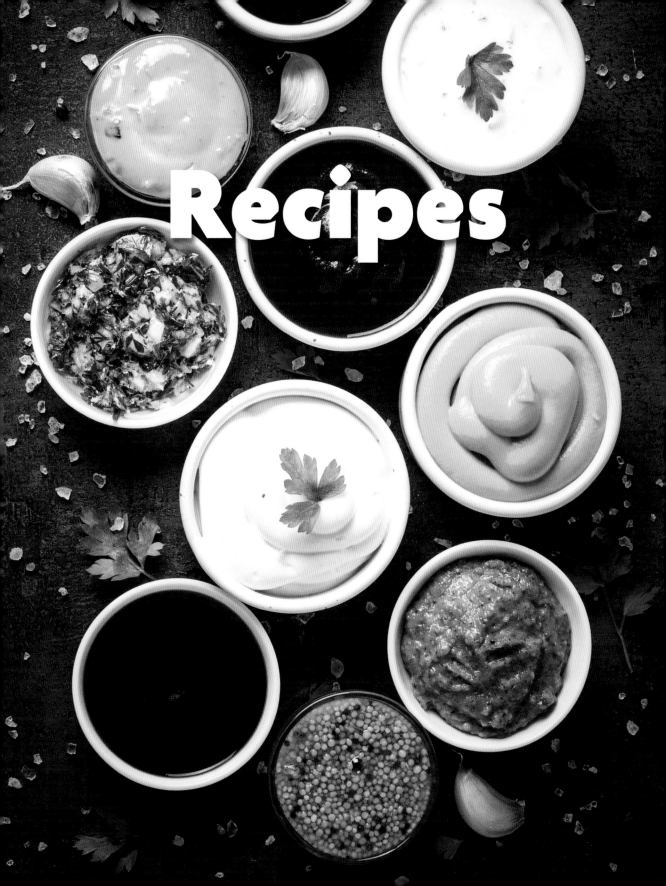

Recipes

CHAPTER 3
Rubs and Marinades

Rubs and marinades are the pregame preparation before the big barbecue show. They're both used to create a dimension of flavor for the proteins during the cooking process.

Rubs

Rubs are normally in a dry form but can also be wet in a paste form.

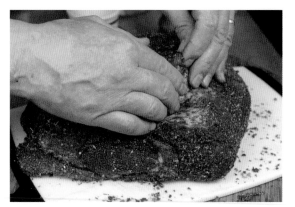

To use a dry rub:

- Pat down protein with a paper towel to remove any surface water.

- Place a tablespoon or so of a neutral oil on the surface of the meat and use your hands to spread the oil for even coverage.

- Lightly shake the rub over the surface (don't cake it on), and use a dry hand to pat or lightly press the rub into the meat.

- Let the meat rest for a few minutes to a few hours before cooking.

Watch the salt content in a dry rub, especially if you're going to add salt to a protein and then let it rest overnight.

Marinades

Marinades are a little different from rubs in that they are usually wet. In addition to providing flavor, they also tenderize proteins via an acid (e.g., vinegar or citrus juice) or enzymes from bacterial cultures (e.g., yogurt or sour cream). Here are some marinating tips:

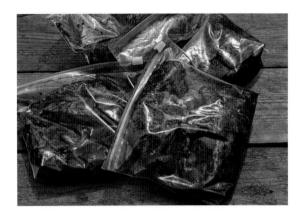

- Marinate for a few hours or overnight to give those tenderizers time to do their work and let the flavor penetrate.

- Discard used marinade to avoid cross contamination and foodborne illnesses.

- If you wish to use some marinade during cooking or in serving, make extra and set some aside. Add in the unused marinade in the cooking process or as a side in serving.

- Zip-top bags are useful for marinating to keep the marinade in contact with all surfaces and ensure the protein is covered. A shallow bowl can work too.

- A time-saving, money-saving, and meal-prep tip: Purchase larger cuts of meats on sale and then portion them down to smaller sizes. Add a marinade to a zip-top bag along with the portioned protein, seal, label, and then freeze. When you're ready to use it, pop the bag in the fridge and while the meat thaws, it marinates at the same time.

Basic Brisket Rub

Sometimes with a brisket, you just want it to shine from that 9-hour-plus smoke. A simple rub like this one is best to accentuate the natural flavor of the brisket and smoke.

Makes: ½ cup | **Serving Size:** 1 teaspoon

¼ cup salt

¼ cup black pepper

2 tablespoons garlic powder

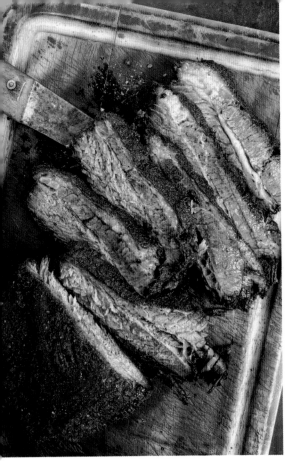

1. Mix all of the ingredients together in a small bowl.

2. The rub is ready to use immediately. Store any excess rub in an airtight container away from heat, light, and moisture. Use stored rub within a couple of months.

> **NUTRITION PER SERVING: Calories:** 3 | **Net Carbohydrates:** 0.4g | **Fat:** 0g | **Protein:** 0.1g | **Carbohydrates:** 0.6g | **Fiber:** 0.2g

Asian Five-Spice Rub

While great on chicken and chicken wings as is, this rub is stunning on pork and pork belly with the addition of 2 teaspoons of salt.

Makes: ½ cup | **Serving Size:** 1 teaspoon

3 tablespoons garlic power

3 tablespoons onion powder

1 tablespoon five-spice powder

1½ teaspoons ground ginger

1½ teaspoons black pepper

1. Mix all of the ingredients together in a small bowl.

2. The rub is ready to use immediately. Store any excess rub in an airtight container away from heat, light, and moisture. Use stored rub within a couple of months.

> **NUTRITION PER SERVING: Calories:** 8 | **Net Carbohydrates:** 1.4g | **Fat:** 0.1g | **Protein:** 0.3g | **Carbohydrates:** 1.8g | **Fiber:** 0.4g

Beef Rub

Brisket, beef ribs, steak, sirloin roast! Sprinkle on, let rest, then pop it in the smoker.

Makes: ⅔ cup | **Serving Size:** 1 teaspoon

4 tablespoons brown Swerve

1 tablespoon ancho chili powder

½ teaspoon ground cayenne pepper

½ teaspoon ground cumin

1 tablespoon paprika

1 teaspoon onion powder

1 teaspoon garlic powder

½ teaspoon mustard powder

1 teaspoon ground nutmeg

½ tablespoon salt

½ teaspoon black pepper

1. Mix all of the ingredients together in a small bowl.

2. The rub is ready to use immediately. Store any excess rub in an airtight container away from heat, light, and moisture. Use within a couple of weeks. Stored rub may clump due to the sweetener used; this is normal. Break apart the clumps with either your fingers or a fork before using.

NUTRITION PER SERVING: **Calories:** 3 | **Net Carbohydrates:** 0.3g | **Fat:** 0.1g | **Protein:** 0.1g | **Carbohydrates:** 0.5g | **Fiber:** 0.2g

Pork Belly Rub

Toss some pork belly cubes in this rub before smoking. Serve with a vinegar sauce for nice flavor contrast.

Makes: ⅓ cup | **Serving Size:** 1 teaspoon

2 teaspoons dried onion

2 teaspoons dried garlic

¼ teaspoon ground cayenne pepper

¼ teaspoon citric acid

1 teaspoon mustard powder

1 tablespoon granular Swerve

2 tablespoons brown Swerve

2 teaspoons salt

½ teaspoon black pepper

1. Mix all of the ingredients together in a small bowl.

2. The rub is ready to use immediately. Store any excess rub in an airtight container away from heat, light, and moisture. Use within a couple of weeks. Stored rub may clump due to the sweetener used; this is normal. Break apart the clumps with either your fingers or a fork before using.

NUTRITION PER SERVING: Calories: 4 | **Net Carbohydrates:** 0.6g | **Fat:** 0.1g | **Protein:** 0.2g | **Carbohydrates:** 0.7g | **Fiber:** 0.1g

Espresso Rub

Looking to try something a little different? Try this rub on a beef or lamb roast and let it sit overnight. This allows the flavors to mellow and comingle before low and slow cooking.

Makes: 6 tablespoons | **Serving Size:** 1 teaspoon

2 tablespoons ground espresso

2 tablespoons smoked paprika

1 teaspoon dried garlic

1 teaspoon dried onion

2 tablespoons brown Swerve

1 teaspoon salt

½ teaspoon black pepper

1. Mix all of the ingredients together in a small bowl.

2. The rub is ready to use immediately. Store any excess rub in an airtight container away from heat, light, and moisture. Use within a couple of weeks. Stored rub may clump due to the sweetener used; this is normal. Break apart the clumps with either your fingers or a fork before using.

NUTRITION PER SERVING: Calories: 2 | **Net Carbohydrates:** 0.3g | **Fat:** 0g | **Protein:** 0.1g | **Carbohydrates:** 0.4g | **Fiber:** 0.1g

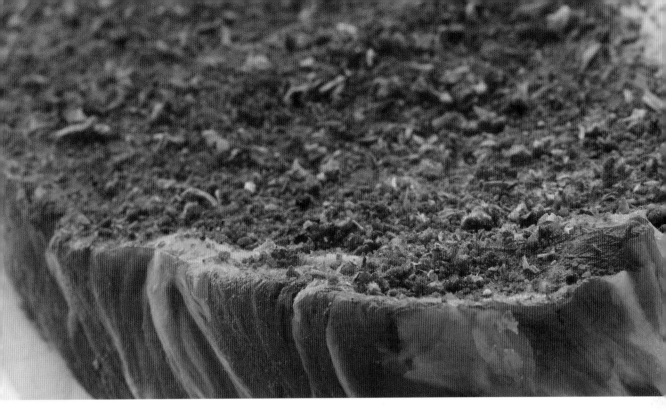

Cajun/Blackened Rub

Packed with flavor and heat. After seasoning your chicken, fish, or seafood with this rub, let it rest for a few hours before cooking. Serve with some grilled vegetables along the Chili Lime Dip (page 90).

Makes: 5½ tablespoons | **Serving Size:** 1 teaspoon

1 tablespoon smoked paprika

2 tablespoons paprika

1 teaspoon dried garlic

1 teaspoon dried onion

½ teaspoon black pepper

2 teaspoons dried thyme

2 teaspoons dried oregano

1 teaspoon ground cayenne pepper

1 teaspoon salt

1. Mix all of the ingredients together in a small bowl.

2. The rub is ready to use immediately. Store any excess rub in an airtight container away from heat, light, and moisture. Use stored rub within a couple of months.

NUTRITION PER SERVING: **Calories:** 6 | **Net Carbohydrates:** 0.6g | **Fat:** 0.2g | **Protein:** 0.3g | **Carbohydrates:** 1.2g | **Fiber:** 0.6g

Fish Rub

Sprinkle on your favorite fish, seafood, or vegetables before grilling. Serve it with Tartar Sauce (page 63).

Makes: 5½ tablespoons | **Serving Size:** 1 teaspoon

1 tablespoon dried basil

½ teaspoon cracked coriander

½ teaspoon red pepper flakes

1 teaspoon onion powder

1 tablespoon dried parsley

1 tablespoon dried tarragon

1 teaspoon granular Swerve

1 (0.8–gram) packet True Lemon

½ teaspoon dried garlic

¼ teaspoon citric acid

¼ teaspoon amchoor powder (optional)

1 teaspoon salt

1. Mix all of the ingredients together well in a small bowl.

2. The rub is ready to use immediately. Store any excess rub in an airtight container away from heat, light, and moisture. Use within a few weeks. Stored rub may clump due to the sweetener used; this is normal. Break apart the clumps with either your fingers or a fork before using.

3. Before using, make sure the rub is well mixed as the heavier spices sink to the bottom.

> **NUTRITION PER SERVING: Calories:** 3 | **Net Carbohydrates:** 0.3g | **Fat:** 0.1g | **Protein:** 0.2g | **Carbohydrates:** 0.5g | **Fiber:** 0.2g

Italian Rub

Lovely on a whole rotisserie grilled chicken or chicken thighs. Try using it in the smoker.

Makes: 6 tablespoons | **Serving Size:** 1 teaspoon

1½ tablespoons dried oregano

1½ tablespoons dried thyme

1 teaspoon dried garlic

2 teaspoons dried rosemary

2 teaspoons chili flakes

1 teaspoon sea salt

2 turns cracked black peppercorns

1. Mix all of the ingredients well in a small bowl.

2. The rub is ready to use immediately. Store excess rub in an airtight container away from heat, light, and moisture. Use stored rub within a couple of months.

> **NUTRITION PER SERVING: Calories:** 10 | **Net Carbohydrates:** 1.2g | **Fat:** 0.3g | **Protein:** 0.4g | **Carbohydrates:** 2.3g | **Fiber:** 1.1g

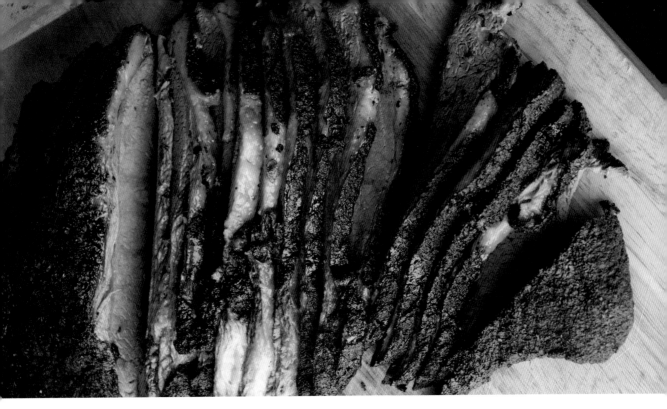

Memphis-Style Rub

A great rub that complements pork shoulder and the dry rib Memphis-Style barbecue on a pit smoker, with flavors that are similar to that of chili seasoning.

Makes: 2½ cups | **Serving Size:** 1 teaspoon

¾ cup brown Swerve

¼ cup granular Swerve or erythritol

½ cup paprika

¼ cup garlic powder

2 tablespoons sea salt

2 tablespoons black pepper

2 tablespoons ground ginger

2 tablespoons onion powder

1 tablespoon dried oregano

2 teaspoons ground thyme

1. Mix all of the ingredients together in small bowl.

2. The rub is ready to use immediately. Store any excess rub in an airtight container away from heat, light, and moisture. Use within a few weeks. Stored rub may clump due to the sweetener used; this is normal. Break apart the clumps with your fingers or a fork before using.

NUTRITION PER SERVING: **Calories:** 3 | **Net Carbohydrates:** 0.4g | **Fat:** 0.1g | **Protein:** 0.1g | **Carbohydrates:** 0.6g | **Fiber:** 0.2g

Sweet Jamaican Jerk Rub

A spicy rub with a hint of sweetness and a little bit of warmth. For a more traditional Jamaican jerk rub, use Scotch bonnet pepper powder for that real spicy kick.

Makes: 5½ tablespoons | **Serving Size:** 1 teaspoon

1 tablespoon ground allspice

4 teaspoons dried thyme

1½ teaspoons ground cinnamon

¾ teaspoon ground cloves

½ teaspoon garlic powder

1½ teaspoons ground ginger

1½ teaspoons ground nutmeg

¾ teaspoon powdered serrano pepper

½ teaspoon citric acid (optional)

2 teaspoons brown Swerve

1 teaspoon sea salt

¼ teaspoon black pepper

1. Mix all of the ingredients well in a small bowl.

2. The rub is ready to use immediately. Store any excess rub in an airtight container away from heat, light, and moisture. Use within a few weeks. Stored rub may clump due to the sweetener used; this is normal. Break apart the clumps with your fingers or a fork before using.

NUTRITION PER SERVING: **Calories:** 5 | **Net Carbohydrates:** 0.6g | **Fat:** 0.2g | **Protein:** 0.1g | **Carbohydrates:** 1.1g | **Fiber:** 0.5g

Mole Rub

Use this earthy Mexican-inspired rub that uses cocoa powder on pork and chicken with some lime juice. Serve with a side of fresh Guacamole (page 115).

Makes: 5½ tablespoons | **Serving Size:** 1 teaspoon

2 tablespoons Dutch-processed dark cocoa

¼ teaspoon ground cinnamon

1 teaspoon garlic powder

1 teaspoon chipotle chili powder

1 tablespoon ancho chili powder

1½ teaspoons sea salt

1 teaspoon dried thyme

1. Mix all of the ingredients together in a small bowl.

2. The rub is ready to use immediately. Store any excess rub in an airtight container away from heat, light, and moisture. Use stored rub within a couple of months.

NUTRITION PER SERVING: Calories: 4 | **Net Carbohydrates:** 0.4g | **Fat:** 0.2g | **Protein:** 0.2g | **Carbohydrates:** 0.8g | **Fiber:** 0.4g

Moroccan Rub

This recipe started when I was inspired to use cinnamon in a rub. As I was pulling out spices from the pantry, I realized that these spices are characteristic of Moroccan cuisine. Try this rub on beef. It goes great on lamb too!

Makes: ¼ cup | **Serving Size:** 1 teaspoon

4 teaspoons paprika

1 teaspoon cracked coriander seed

1 teaspoon ground cinnamon

1¼ teaspoons ground cumin

¼ teaspoon ground cloves

¼ teaspoon ground ginger

2 teaspoons sea salt

½ teaspoon black pepper

1. Mix all of the ingredients together in a small bowl.

2. The rub is ready to use immediately. Store any extra rub in an airtight container away from heat, light, and moisture. Use stored rub within a couple of months.

NUTRITION PER SERVING: Calories: 2 | **Net Carbohydrates:** 0.3g | **Fat:** 0.1g | **Protein:** 0.1g | **Carbohydrates:** 0.5g | **Fiber:** 0.2g

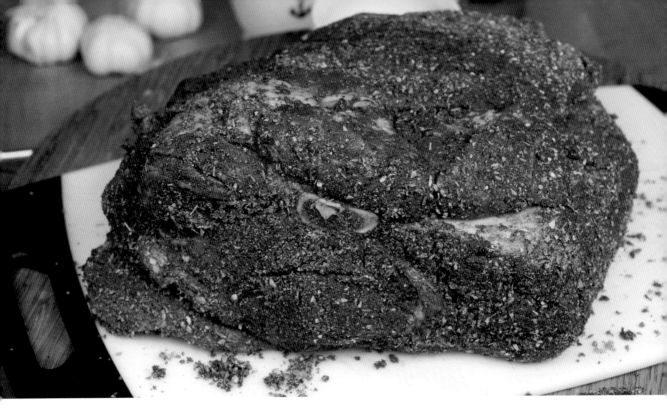

Pork Rub

A little on the sweeter side, this rub loves pork and pork ribs. Try it on some chicken wings too!

Makes: about ½ cup | **Serving Size:** 1 teaspoon

2 tablespoons sea salt

1 tablespoon brown Swerve

1 tablespoon granular Swerve

1 tablespoon ancho chili powder

2 tablespoons paprika

2 teaspoons dried garlic

2 teaspoons black pepper

1. Mix all of the ingredients together in a small bowl.

2. The rub is ready to use immediately. Store any excess rub in an airtight container away from heat, light, and moisture. Use within a few weeks. Stored rub may clump due to the sweetener used; this is normal. Break apart the clumps with your fingers or a fork before using.

NUTRITION PER SERVING: Calories: 4 | **Net Carbohydrates:** 0.4g | **Fat:** 0.1g | **Protein:** 0.2g | **Carbohydrates:** 0.8g | **Fiber:** 0.4g

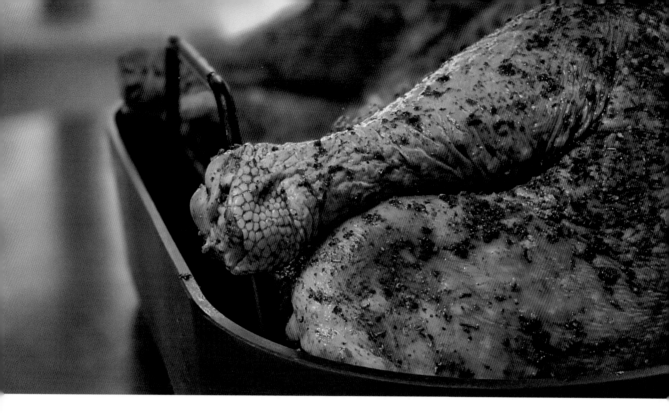

Poultry Rub

A savory poultry rub for chicken and turkey. Brush on the Cranberry Barbecue Sauce (page 71) during the last 10 or 15 minutes of cooking.

Makes: ½ cup | **Serving Size:** 1 teaspoon

4 teaspoons garlic powder

4 teaspoons onion powder

¼ cup paprika

2 tablespoons sea salt

2 teaspoons black pepper

1. Mix all of the ingredients together in a small bowl.

2. The rub is ready to use immediately. Store any excess rub in an airtight container away from heat, light, and moisture. Use stored rub within a couple of months.

NUTRITION PER SERVING: **Calories:** 7 | **Net Carbohydrates:** 0.9g | **Fat:** 0.2g | **Protein:** 0.3g | **Carbohydrates:** 1.5g | **Fiber:** 0.6g

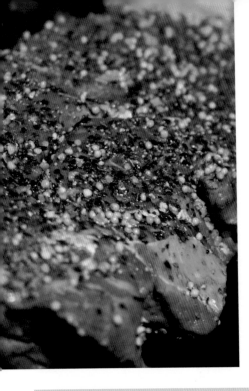

Steak Rub

Sprinkle on top of steaks before they hit the grill. After grilling, choose your favorite compound butter to serve on top.

Makes: ¼ cup | **Serving Size:** 1 teaspoon

2 teaspoons garlic powder

2 teaspoons cracked coriander seed

1 teaspoon chili flakes

2½ teaspoons cracked black peppercorns

3½ teaspoons sea salt

1. Mix all of the ingredients together in a small bowl.

2. The rub is ready to use immediately. Store any excess rub in an airtight container away from heat, light, and moisture. Use stored rub within a couple of months.

NUTRITION PER SERVING: Calories: 4 | **Net Carbohydrates:** 0.7g | **Fat:** 0.1g | **Protein:** 0.2g | **Carbohydrates:** 1.0g | **Fiber:** 0.3g

Tex–Mex Rub

Where spicy, sweet, smoky, and tangy collide. So good, you'll want to use it on everything. Serve it with Pico de Gallo (page 117) and/or fresh Guacamole (page 115).

Makes: 6 tablespoons | **Serving Size:** 1 teaspoon

1 teaspoon ground cumin

1 teaspoon salt

¼ teaspoon black pepper

1 tablespoon dried oregano

3 tablespoons chili powder

1 teaspoon garlic powder

½ teaspoon ground cayenne pepper

1 tablespoon paprika

½ teaspoon chipotle chili powder

1. Mix all of the ingredients together in a small bowl.

2. The rub is ready to use immediately. Store any excess in an airtight container away from heat, light, and moisture. Use stored rub within a couple of months.

NUTRITION PER SERVING: Calories: 7 | **Net Carbohydrates:** 0.6g | **Fat:** 0.3g | **Protein:** 0.3g | **Carbohydrates:** 1.3g | **Fiber:** 0.7g

Tandoori Rub

Popular in Indian cuisine, this spicy rub works well with chicken, lamb, and fish. The cool, creamy contrast of the Tzatziki sauce (page 119) pairs well with this rub.

Makes: 6 tablespoons | **Serving Size:** 1 teaspoon

3 tablespoons paprika

½ teaspoon ground cumin

1 teaspoon ground turmeric

¾ teaspoon ground cayenne pepper

1 teaspoon ground coriander

1 teaspoon ground ginger

½ teaspoon ground nutmeg

1 teaspoon dried garlic

1 teaspoon garam masala

1 teaspoon salt

1. Mix all of the ingredients together in a small bowl.

2. The rub is ready to use immediately. Store any excess rub in an airtight container away from heat, light, and moisture. Use stored rub within a couple of months.

NUTRITION PER SERVING: **Calories:** 8 | **Net Carbohydrates:** 0.6g | **Fat:** 0.2g | **Protein:** 0.2g | **Carbohydrates:** 1.1g | **Fiber:** 0.5g

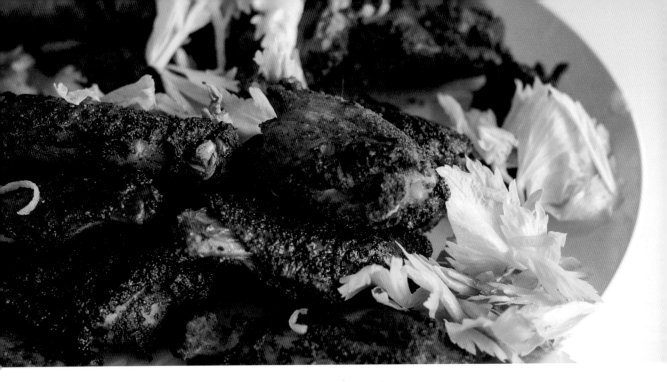

A Rub for Wings

A rub for wings that's great for in the smoker! Try it with the Alabama
White Barbecue Sauce (page 62), it will change your life!

Makes: ¼ cup | **Serving Size:** 1 teaspoon

2 tablespoons paprika

2 tablespoons ancho chili powder

1 teaspoon ground cumin

1 teaspoon onion powder

1 teaspoon garlic powder

1 teaspoon celery seed

½ teaspoon ground cayenne pepper

1 teaspoon salt

1 teaspoon black pepper

1. Mix all of the ingredients together in a small bowl.

2. The rub is ready to use immediately. Store any excess in an airtight container away from
heat, light, and moisture. Use stored rub within a couple of months.

NUTRITION PER SERVING: Calories: 11 | **Net Carbohydrates:** 1g |
Fat: 0.4g | **Protein:** 0.5g | **Carbohydrates:** 2g | **Fiber:** 1g

Annie's Marinade

This is one of my favorite barbecue marinades that my mom makes. She would just effortlessly throw these ingredients together without measuring and then marinate thin beef slices for a couple of hours. It always turned out delicious. It was a little bit of a challenge to get exact amounts! It's great on beef but is absolutely out of this world with thin pork slices. Break out the coals for this one! Serve with a coleslaw made with the Asian Sesame Dip (page 88).

Makes: ¾ cup | **Serving Size:** 1 teaspoon

¼ cup liquid aminos or soy sauce

1 tablespoon Worcestershire sauce

3 tablespoons sugar-free ketchup

1 tablespoon olive oil

2 cloves, crushed

1 tablespoon apple cider vinegar

½ tablespoon grated ginger

2 teaspoons granular Swerve

⅛ teaspoon xanthan gum (optional)

1. Whisk all of the ingredients together in a small bowl.

2. If the Swerve doesn't dissolve, microwave the marinade for about 30 seconds to warm, and whisk. If it's still not fully dissolved, continue heating and whisking until incorporated.

3. If thickening is desired, thicken by sprinkling in xanthan gum over the marinade and whisk in. Heating isn't required.

4. The marinade is ready to use. If not using the marinade immediately, refrigerate in a covered nonreactive vessel such as a glass jar. Use within a couple of days.

NUTRITION PER SERVING: **Calories:** 6 | **Net Carbohydrates:** 0.4g | **Fat:** 0.4g | **Protein:** 0.2g | **Carbohydrates:** 0.4g | **Fiber:** 0g

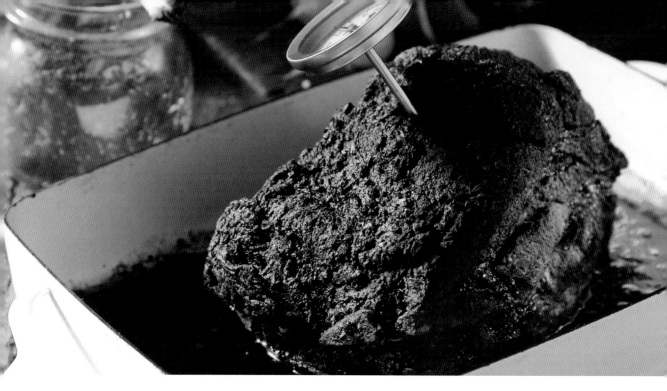

Caribbean Pork Marinade

This marinade is usually used on a pork shoulder or a whole leg. These bold Caribbean flavors work best if the pork marinates overnight.

Makes: 1½ cups | **Serving Size:** 1 teaspoon

2 tablespoons lime juice

2 teaspoons lime zest

8 cloves garlic, peeled and roughly chopped

1 medium onion, roughly chopped

2 teaspoons dried Mexican oregano

1 teaspoon dried thyme

4 teaspoons ground cumin

2 teaspoons paprika

1 teaspoon chipotle chili powder

1 tablespoon sea salt

1½ teaspoons black pepper

5 tablespoons extra-virgin olive oil

1. Add all of the ingredients except the olive oil to a blender, and blend until fine.

2. Once blended, whisk in the olive oil.

3. The marinade will resemble a paste and is ready to use immediately. Make the rub just before you need it and don't store any leftovers.

4. To use, spread the marinade paste over the meat to cover the entire piece.

NUTRITION PER SERVING: Calories: 11 | **Net Carbohydrates:** 0.4g | **Fat:** 0.5g | **Protein:** 0g | **Carbohydrates:** 0.5g | **Fiber:** 0.1g

Citrus Marinade

This citrus marinade is great for chicken and vegetables. It's ideal for chicken, pork, and lamb skewers. Just marinate inch-cubed pieces of protein for a couple of hours, then place them on a skewer before grilling. Serve with Tzatziki sauce (page 119).

This marinade can be used as a salad dressing too! Just add about ½ to 1 teaspoon of sweetener for balance.

Makes: ¾ cup | **Serving Size:** 1 teaspoon

1 tablespoon dried oregano

1 tablespoon dried dill

1½ tablespoons dried rosemary

1 teaspoon dried thyme

4 cloves garlic, crushed

2 teaspoons salt

½ cup lemon juice

zest of 1 lemon

¼ cup olive oil

1. Mix the spices, including the salt, with the lemon juice and zest in a small bowl.

2. Whisk in the olive oil until incorporated well.

3. Let the marinade sit for about 15 minutes for the dried spices to hydrate before using.

4. The marinade is ready to use. If not using the marinade immediately, refrigerate in a covered nonreactive vessel such as a glass jar. Use within a couple of days.

NUTRITION PER SERVING: **Calories:** 12 | **Net Carbohydrates:** 0.4g | **Fat:** 1.3g | **Protein:** 0.1g | **Carbohydrates:** 0.5g | **Fiber:** 0.1g

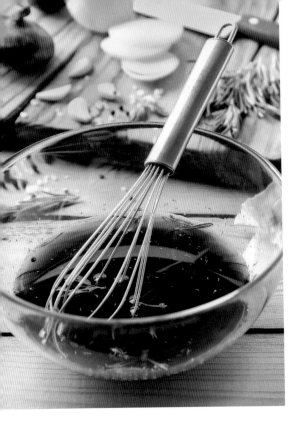

Garlic Soy Marinade

Similar to a teriyaki sauce with infused garlic and onion to add that hint of flavor. Try it with fish and serve with a side of the Wasabi Aioli (page 86)

Makes: 1 cup | **Serving Size:** 1 tablespoon

1 tablespoon avocado oil

½ cup chopped onion

3 cloves garlic, lightly crushed

⅓ cup liquid aminos

1 cup water

⅛ teaspoon liquid monk fruit

2 tablespoons brown Swerve

⅛ teaspoon xanthan gum (optional)

1. Add the oil to a medium saucepan over medium-high heat. Once hot, add the chopped onion and sauté for 5 minutes, until softened.

2. Add the garlic and quickly sauté for about 15 seconds.

3. Add the liquid aminos, water, and monk fruit. Whisk in the Swerve.

4. Bring the mixture to a boil.

5. Turn down the heat and simmer for 10 minutes.

6. Remove from heat and let cool.

7. Strain out the garlic and onion.

8. If desired, thicken by sprinkling xanthan gum on top and whisk in.

9. The marinade is ready to use. If not using the marinade immediately, refrigerate in a covered nonreactive vessel such as a glass jar. Use within a couple of days.

NUTRITION PER SERVING: Calories: 11 | **Net Carbohydrates:** 0.3g | **Fat:** 0.9g | **Protein:** 0.6g | **Carbohydrates:** 0.3g | **Fiber:** 0g

Persian Chicken Marinade

The full-fat sour cream tenderizes and seals in the juices of the chicken, as well as imparts a delicious tanginess, along with the lemon juice. To best bring out these bright flavors, marinate your chicken overnight and cook it over coals.

Makes: ½ cup | Serving Size: 2 teaspoons

¼ teaspoon saffron powder (about 15 to 20 ground saffron strands)

½ teaspoon sea salt, divided if necessary

2 tablespoons hot water

½ cup full-fat sour cream

2 tablespoons lemon juice

¼ teaspoon black pepper

¼ cup sliced onion

1. If you are using saffron strands, grind them to a powder with a mortar and pestle. Then, in a small bowl, combine your resulting saffron powder with half the salt.

2. Transfer the saffron powder to a ramekin or a small bowl and add the hot water to let the saffron "bloom" for about 10 minutes.

3. Meanwhile, in another bowl, mix the sour cream, lemon juice, black pepper, and the remaining salt (or the full amount if you used the saffron powder to start).

4. Whisk the saffron water into the sour cream mixture.

5. Stir in the sliced onions.

6. The marinade is ready to use. If not using the marinade immediately, refrigerate in a covered nonreactive vessel such as a glass jar. Use within a couple of days.

7. Before barbecuing, discard the onions.

NUTRITION PER SERVING:* Calories: 20 | Net Carbohydrates: 0.6g | Fat: 1.9g | Protein: 0.2g | Carbohydrates: 0.6g | Fiber: 0g

*Onion is not included in the nutrition values since it's used to infuse flavor and is discarded.

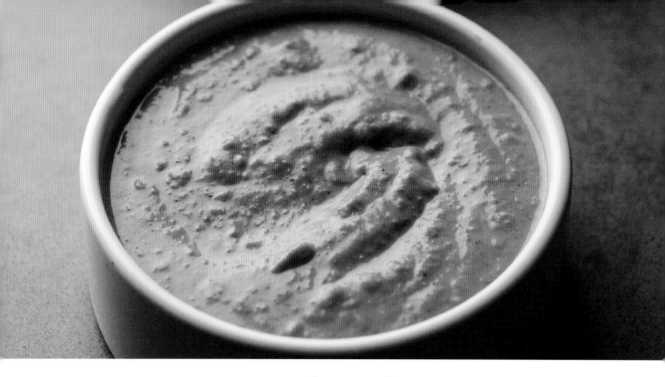

Tandoori Marinade

Great with chicken. Try it with chicken wings and let it marinate overnight in the fridge. For a spicier tandoori, increase the cayenne powder to a teaspoon. Serve with Tzatziki (page 119) for a nice contrast.

Makes: 1¼ cups | **Serving Size:** 2 teaspoons

1 teaspoon ground coriander seed

1 teaspoon ground cumin seed

½ teaspoon ground turmeric

¾ teaspoon ground cayenne pepper

½ tablespoon ancho chili powder

1 tablespoon garam masala

2 tablespoons paprika

2 teaspoons sea salt

1 cup full-fat yogurt or full-fat sour cream

1 tablespoon lemon juice

2 cloves garlic, minced

2 teaspoons minced ginger

1. Mix the dry spices together in a small bowl and set aside.

2. In a separate medium bowl, mix the yogurt, lemon juice, garlic, and ginger.

3. Whisk the dry spices into the yogurt mixture and let sit for about 5 minutes before using

4. The marinade is ready to use. If not using the marinade immediately, refrigerate in a covered nonreactive vessel such as a glass jar. Use within a couple of days.

NUTRITION PER SERVING: Calories: 13 | **Net Carbohydrates:** 0.6g | **Fat:** 0.6g | **Protein:** 1g | **Carbohydrates:** 0.9g | **Fiber:** 0.3g

Shawarma Marinade

Shawarma originates from Middle Eastern cooking and consists of stacking and cooking thin slices of lamb on a vertical rotisserie. While it can be challenging to find a vertical rotisserie to cook authentic Shawarma, I took inspiration from some of the seasonings used for a marinade. The flavors really shine through when using thin slices of meats. Feel free to use it on lamb, but this marinade does wonders for chicken. After marinating (best overnight), pop the chicken onto some skewers and grill.

Makes: ½ cup | **Serving Size:** 1 teaspoon

¾ teaspoon dried oregano

½ teaspoon ground cinnamon

½ teaspoon coriander powder

½ teaspoon ground cumin

⅛ teaspoon ground turmeric

½ teaspoon ground ginger

2 teaspoons paprika

2 cloves garlic, minced

1 teaspoon sea salt

½ teaspoon black pepper

1 tablespoon brown Swerve

2 tablespoons hot water

3 tablespoons lemon juice

¼ cup extra-virgin olive oil

1. Mix the dried spices, garlic, salt, and black pepper in a small bowl. Set aside.

2. In a separate bowl, dissolve the Swerve in the hot water while stirring.

3. Once dissolved, add the lemon juice and the olive oil.

4. Whisk the dried spices into the liquid.

5. Let the marinade rest for a few minutes before using.

6. The marinade is ready to use. If not using the marinade immediately, refrigerate in a covered nonreactive vessel such as a glass jar. Use within a couple of days.

NUTRITION PER SERVING: **Calories:** 22 | **Net Carbohydrates:** 0.4g | **Fat:** 2.4g | **Protein:** 0.1g | **Carbohydrates:** 0.6g | **Fiber:** 0.2g

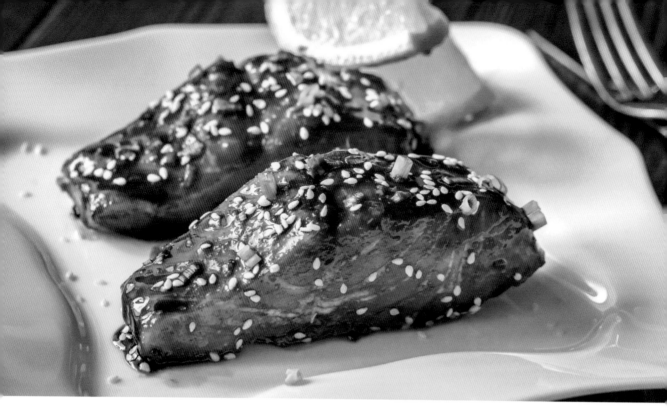

Teriyaki Marinade

A traditional teriyaki marinade. Use it to marinate chicken,
duck, beef, or pork, then pop it on the grill.

Makes: 1 cup | **Serving Size:** 1 teaspoon

½ cup liquid aminos or soy sauce

½ cup rice vinegar

¼ cup granular Swerve

¼ teaspoon xanthan gum (optional)

1. Whisk all of the ingredients together.

2. If the Swerve doesn't dissolve, microwave the sauce for about 30 seconds to warm, and whisk. If it's still not fully dissolved, continue heating and whisking until incorporated.

3. If desired, sprinkle and then whisk in xanthan gum to thicken.

4. The marinade is ready to use. If not using the marinade immediately, refrigerate in a covered nonreactive vessel such as a glass jar. Use within a couple of days.

NUTRITION PER SERVING: Calories: 3 | **Net Carbohydrates:** 0.2g | **Fat:** 0g | **Protein:** 0.3g | **Carbohydrates:** 0.2g | **Fiber:** 0g

CHAPTER 4

Condiments and Sauces

What's a barbecue without those condiments and sauces? Whether it's mustard on a hot dog, ketchup on a burger, or barbecue sauce on a rack of ribs, condiments are always present at barbecues. They bring another dimension to your favorite barbecued foods.

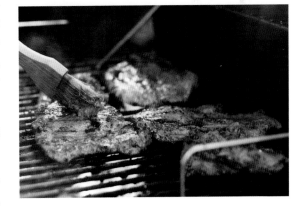

Here are a few ideas on using condiments and sauces in different ways:

- Brush on while grilling or during the last hour or half hour of a smoke to let the sauce caramelize.

- Serve on the side at the table, perhaps in a condiment squeeze bottle.

- Mix in a couple of tablespoons with pulled meats such as pork, beef, or chicken.

- Use as a dipping sauce.

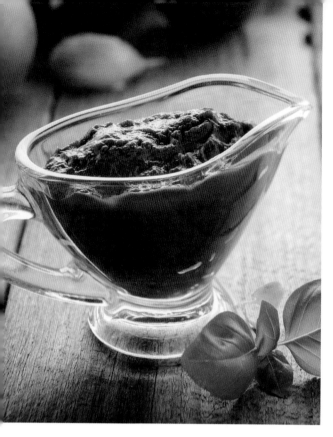

Ketchup

There's nothing like having your own homemade ketchup, a base for many other sauces. If you like it tangier, add a little more apple cider vinegar.

Makes: 3½ cups | **Serving Size:** 1 tablespoon

1 tablespoon avocado or olive oil

½ cup chopped onion

1 clove garlic, crushed

1 (26-ounce) can crushed tomatoes

6 tablespoons white vinegar

1 tablespoon apple cider vinegar

1 tablespoon granular Swerve

½ can tomato paste

¾ teaspoon ground allspice

½ teaspoon ground cloves

2 teaspoons sea salt

1. Add the oil to a medium saucepan over medium-high heat. Once warm, add the chopped onion and sauté for about 2 to 3 minutes, until softened.

2. Add the garlic and quickly sauté for about 15 seconds.

3. Mix in all of the remaining ingredients and cook for about 45 to 50 minutes, stirring occasionally to reduce the liquid.

4. Blend with a stick blender in the pot to mix and to chop up chunks.

5. Lower the heat and simmer for about 30 minutes or to desired thickness, whisking the liquid occasionally to prevent sticking.

6. Remove from heat and let cool slightly before transferring to a glass or plastic container. Glass sauce or plastic condiment bottles are always convenient to use.

7. Refrigerate for up to 2 weeks.

NUTRITION PER SERVING: **Calories:** 7 | **Net Carbohydrates:** 0.6g | **Fat:** 0.3g | **Protein:** 0.2g | **Carbohydrates:** 1g | **Fiber:** 0.4g

Spicy Ketchup

A balanced ketchup with a little bit of heat, this is a great side condiment but also a good base for red barbecue sauces.

Makes: 3½ cups | **Serving Size:** 1 tablespoon

2 tablespoons brown Swerve

½ teaspoon onion powder

½ teaspoon garlic powder

1 teaspoon ground cayenne pepper

½ teaspoon ground allspice

¼ teaspoon ground cloves

⅛ teaspoon ground cinnamon

2 teaspoons salt

1 (26-ounce) can crushed tomatoes

4½ tablespoons apple cider vinegar

½ tablespoon apple cider vinegar (optional)

1. Mix the Swerve, onion powder, garlic powder, cayenne, allspice, cloves, cinnamon, and salt in a small bowl.

2. In a saucepan over medium-high heat, add the crushed tomatoes and apple cider vinegar.

3. Whisk in the spice mix. Bring the sauce to the beginnings of a boil, about 5 minutes, and then reduce the heat to medium low.

4. Continue to heat for 15 to 20 minutes to reduce the water, whisking occasionally to prevent clumping. For a thicker ketchup, continue to reduce the water for an additional 30 to 35 minutes.

5. If you like a tangier ketchup, whisk in an additional ½ tablespoon of apple cider vinegar after cooking.

6. Transfer the ketchup to jars and store in the fridge for up to 2 weeks.

NUTRITION PER SERVING: **Calories:** 5 | **Net Carbohydrates:** 0.9g | **Fat:** 0.1g | **Protein:** 0.3g | **Carbohydrates:** 1.2g | **Fiber:** 0.3g

Barbecue Sauce

An all-round good barbecue sauce that's just a little sweet, use this for burgers, frankfurter hot dogs, chicken, and ribs.

Makes: about ½ cup | **Serving Size:** 1 tablespoon

½ cup sugar-free ketchup

1½ tablespoons brown Swerve

⅛ teaspoon ground cayenne pepper

¼ teaspoon chipotle chili powder

¾ teaspoon garlic powder

¼ teaspoon onion powder

¼ teaspoon maple extract

1 teaspoon sea salt

1. Whisk all of the ingredients in a small saucepan over medium heat for about 10 minutes, until the sweetener is dissolved.

2. Let cool and then transfer to a covered glass jar. Store in the fridge for up to 2 weeks.

NUTRITION PER SERVING: Calories: 7 | **Net Carbohydrates:** 1.3g | **Fat:** 0g | **Protein:** 0.1g | **Carbohydrates:** 1.4g | **Fiber:** 0.1g

Chipotle Chili Barbecue Sauce

A thick, rich, smoky sauce with a touch of heat.

Makes: 3½ cups | **Serving Size:** 2 tablespoons

1 tablespoon avocado oil

2 cloves garlic, minced

2 cups sugar-free ketchup

1 (6.55-ounce) can chipotle chilies with adobo sauce

2½ tablespoons lime juice

1 teaspoon brown Swerve

½ teaspoon citric acid

½ teaspoon sea salt

1. Heat the avocado oil in a saucepan over medium heat.

2. Once warm, quickly sauté the garlic in the avocado oil for 30 seconds, until fragrant.

3. Add the remaining ingredients and mix.

4. Bring just up to a boil, mix well, and then turn off the heat.

5. Blend with a stick blender to break down chilies, and blend until smooth.

6. Transfer to a jar and store in the fridge for up to 2 weeks.

NUTRITION PER SERVING: Calories: 19 | **Net Carbohydrates:** 1.3g | **Fat:** 0.5g | **Protein:** 0g | **Carbohydrates:** 1.3g | **Fiber:** 0g

Kansas-Inspired Barbecue Sauce

A balance of sweet from the molasses-like influence and savory from this tomato-based sauce that Kansas is known for.

Makes: 4 cups | **Serving Size:** 1 tablespoon

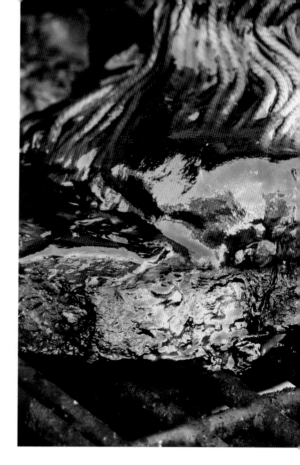

½ teaspoon chili flakes

1 teaspoon ground cayenne pepper

1 teaspoon garlic powder

1 teaspoon onion powder

1 teaspoon smoked paprika

5 tablespoons brown Swerve

2 teaspoons sea salt

1 teaspoon black pepper

1 (26-ounce) can crushed tomatoes

6 tablespoons apple cider vinegar

1 tablespoon Worcestershire sauce

2 tablespoons butter (optional)

1. Mix the dried spices, Swerve, salt, and black pepper together in a small bowl. Set aside.

2. In a saucepan, mix the crushed tomatoes, apple cider vinegar, and Worcestershire sauce.

3. Whisk in the dried seasoning mix.

4. Over medium heat, stir occasionally as the sauce comes to a boil, 5 to 7 minutes.

5. Bring the heat down to low and simmer for about 15 minutes.

6. Remove from heat and stir in the butter, if desired.

7. Let cool, transfer into glass jars and store in the fridge for up to 2 weeks.

NUTRITION PER SERVING: Calories: 8 | **Net Carbohydrates:** 0.8g | **Fat:** 0.4g | **Protein:** 0.2g | **Carbohydrates:** 1.1g | **Fiber:** 0.3g

Whiskey Barbecue Sauce

A tangy sauce with a hit of whiskey. Ribs were made for this sauce.

Makes: 2 cups | **Serving Size:** 1 tablespoon

1 tablespoon avocado oil

2 cloves garlic, minced

½ medium onion, chopped

1 cup sugar-free ketchup

1 tablespoon tomato paste

2 teaspoons Worcestershire sauce

½ cup whiskey

2 tablespoons brown Swerve

1½ teaspoons hot sauce

¾ teaspoon sea salt

½ teaspoon black pepper

1. Heat the avocado oil in a saucepan over medium heat.

2. Once the oil is hot, add the onion and sauté for 2 minutes, until soft and translucent.

3. Add the garlic and quickly sauté for 30 seconds, until fragrant.

4. Add the remaining ingredients and mix.

5. Bring the sauce just to a boil.

6. Turn down the heat and simmer for 15 to 20 minutes.

7. Blend with a stick blender to break down the onion and garlic until smooth.

8. Transfer to a glass jar and store in the fridge for up to 2 weeks.

NUTRITION PER SERVING: **Calories:** 17 | **Net Carbohydrates:** 0.9g |
Fat: 0.4g | **Protein:** 0.1g | **Carbohydrates:** 1.0g | **Fiber:** 0.1g

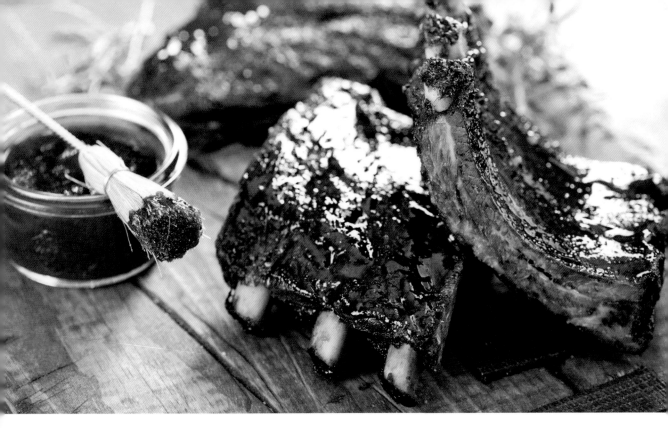

Sweet Hickory Barbecue Sauce

This is for those who like their barbecue sauces sweet. Slather on
chicken or on that rack of ribs, or toss in with pulled pork.

Makes: 1½ cups | **Serving Size:** 1 tablespoon

1 cup sugar–free ketchup

1 cup brown Swerve

½ teaspoon garlic powder

1 teaspoon onion powder

1 teaspoon salt

1½ teaspoons hickory liquid smoke

2 teaspoons Worcestershire sauce

1 tablespoon beef bone broth powder

½ teaspoon balsamic vinegar

¼ teaspoon liquid stevia

1. Whisk all of the ingredients in a small saucepan over medium heat for about 10 minutes,
until the sweetener is dissolved.

2. Let cool, transfer to glass jars, and store in the fridge for up to 2 weeks.

> **NUTRITION PER SERVING: Calories:** 4 | **Net Carbohydrates:** 0.9g
> | **Fat:** 0g | **Protein:** 0g | **Carbohydrates:** 0.9g | **Fiber:** 0g

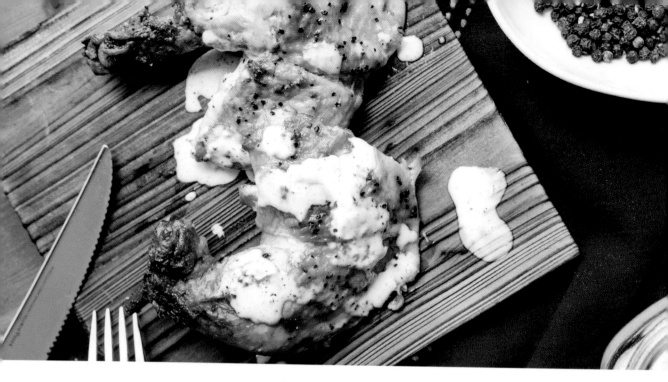

Alabama White Barbecue Sauce

A light, creamy sauce with flavor. First created by Big Bob Gibson in upstate Alabama in 1925, it uses mayonnaise as a base rather than the usual tomato sauce base. It is truly a treat! Try it with wings rubbed in the A Rub for Wings recipe (page 46).

Makes: 1 cup | **Serving Size:** 1 tablespoon

1 cup mayonnaise

2 tablespoons apple cider vinegar

½ teaspoon prepared horseradish

¾ teaspoon salt

¼ teaspoon black pepper

1. Whisk all of the ingredients together in a small bowl.

2. Let sit for 15 minutes before using.

3. Cover and store in the fridge for up to 2 weeks.

NUTRITION PER SERVING: **Calories:** 95 | **Net Carbohydrates:** 0.1g | **Fat:** 10g | **Protein:** 0.1g | **Carbohydrates:** 0.1g | **Fiber:** 0g

Tartar Sauce

This is not your usual tartar sauce, it's got a little extra kick from the added horseradish. Slather it on that grilled or smoked salmon with a Fish Rub (page 38). Goes great with fish, seafood, and chicken.

Makes: 1 cup | **Serving Size:** 2 teaspoons

1 cup mayonnaise

2 tablespoons finely diced dill pickles

2 teaspoons pickle juice

1 teaspoon horseradish

½ teaspoon confectioner's Swerve

½ teaspoon dried dill

½ teaspoon sea salt

¼ teaspoon cracked black peppercorns

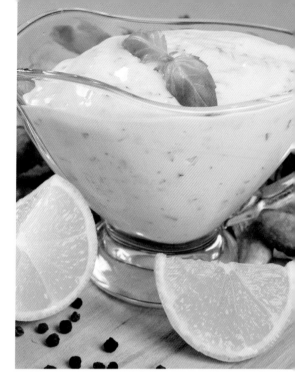

1. Mix all of the ingredients together in a small bowl and let sit for an hour before using.

2. Store sauce in a glass jar in the fridge for up to 2 weeks.

NUTRITION PER SERVING: **Calories:** 64 | **Net Carbohydrates:** 0.3g | **Fat:** 7g | **Protein:** 0.1g | **Carbohydrates:** 0.3g | **Fiber:** 0g

Chicken Sauce

A very simple and incredibly popular condiment, this sweet, creamy rendition of mayonnaise feels almost sinful with chicken and pairs well with salty foods. Use a mayonnaise base that doesn't include lemon.

Makes: 1 cup | **Serving Size:** 1 tablespoon

1 cup mayonnaise

1 teaspoon confectioner's Swerve

1. In a small bowl, add the mayonnaise and whisk in the Swerve. Let sit for about 15 to 30 minutes before enjoying.

2. Store sauce in a glass jar in the fridge for up to 2 weeks.

NUTRITION PER SERVING: **Calories:** 94 | **Net Carbohydrates:** 0.1g | **Fat:** 10.3g | **Protein:** 0.1g | **Carbohydrates:** 0.1g | **Fiber:** 0g

"Fry" Sauce

A creamy, slightly tangy condiment that works well on salty foods. Bring on the hot dogs!

Makes: ¾ cup | **Serving Size:** 1 tablespoon

½ cup mayonnaise

¼ cup sugar–free ketchup

¾ teaspoon paprika

¼ teaspoon confectioner's Swerve

1 teaspoon apple cider vinegar

½ teaspoon salt

1. Whisk all of the ingredients together in a small bowl and let sit for at least 15 minutes before using.

2. Store sauce in a glass jar in the fridge for up to 2 weeks.

> **NUTRITION PER SERVING: Calories:** 48 | **Net Carbohydrates:** 0.4g | **Fat:** 5.2g | **Protein:** 0.1g | **Carbohydrates:** 0.4g | **Fiber:** 0g

Burger Sauce

Reminiscent of those specialty sauces from burger houses, this one is inspired by that flavor when ketchup, mayonnaise, and relish are all combined on a burger. The result? You'll have to try it yourself! You won't want burgers without this sauce.

Makes: 1¼ cup | **Serving Size:** 1 tablespoon

¼ cup finely chopped dill pickle

2 teaspoons sugar–free ketchup

1 cup mayonnaise

½ teaspoon paprika

½ teaspoon salt

2 teaspoons pickle brine

1 teaspoon dried onion

1. Whisk all of the ingredients together in a small bowl and let sit for about 15 minutes before enjoying.

2. Store in a covered glass jar in the fridge for up to 2 weeks.

> **NUTRITION PER SERVING: Calories:** 76 | **Net Carbohydrates:** 0.3g | **Fat:** 8.2g | **Protein:** 0.1g | **Carbohydrates:** 0.4g | **Fiber:** 0.1g

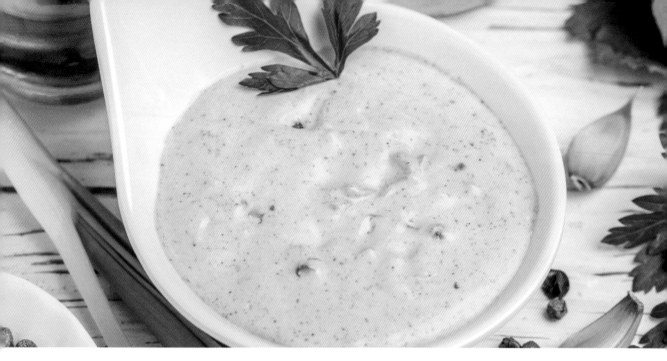

Louisiana Remoulade

Bring on the grilled fish and seafood! The remoulade sauce originated from France and the Cajun community in Louisiana spiced it up a little to make it their own. Here, I created a remoulade with some heat from the hot sauce and cayenne, plus other elements that complement fish and seafood, such as garlic, lemon, and dill. Serve this sauce alongside fish or seafood using the Cajun/Blackened Rub (page 37).

Makes: 1 cup | **Serving Size:** 1 tablespoon

1 cup mayonnaise

1 teaspoon sugar–free ketchup

1 teaspoon cayenne pepper hot sauce

1 teaspoon Worcestershire sauce

2 teaspoons lemon juice

½ teaspoon mustard powder

2 teaspoons paprika

1 teaspoon dried dill

½ teaspoon ground cayenne pepper

½ teaspoon garlic powder

½ teaspoon sea salt

2 turns cracked black peppercorns

1 cornichon pickle, chopped (optional)

1. Whisk all of the ingredients together in a small bowl and let sit for about 15 minutes before enjoying.

2. Store sauce in a glass jar in the fridge for up to 2 weeks.

NUTRITION PER SERVING: **Calories:** 96 | **Net Carbohydrates:** 0.3g | **Fat:** 10.4g | **Protein:** 0.2g | **Carbohydrates:** 0.5g | **Fiber:** 0.2g

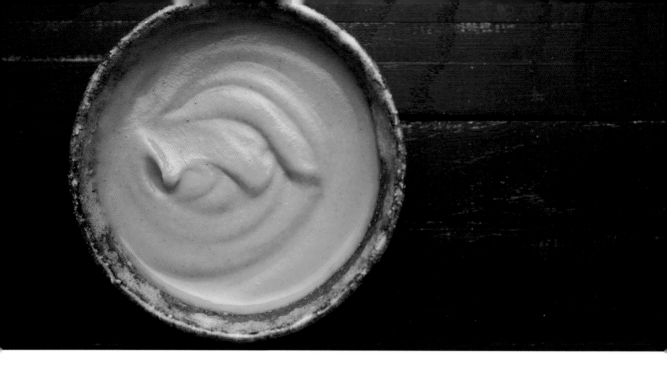

Yellow Mustard

Move the generic yellow prepared mustard over. It is always seen at barbecues, when a homemade mustard is simple to make and has a little more kick than the store-bought variety.

Makes: 1 cup | **Serving Size:** 2 tablespoons

½ cup yellow mustard seeds

¼ cup white vinegar

¾ cup filtered water

½ teaspoon mustard powder

½ teaspoon salt

1 tablespoon pickle brine

¼ cup water

1 tablespoon white vinegar

1 teaspoon granular Swerve

¼ teaspoon ground turmeric

1. Place the mustard seeds, vinegar, and water in a covered jar and let sit in a cool, dark place for 24 to 48 hours.

2. Transfer the mixture to a blender and add in the remaining ingredients.

3. Blend until thoroughly mixed and desired consistency is reached.

4. Let rest for at least 2 hours before serving, though it's best after 24 hours.

5. Store the mustard in a glass jar in the fridge for up to a month.

NUTRITION PER SERVING: **Calories:** 11 | **Net Carbohydrates:** 0.3g | **Fat:** 0.7g | **Protein:** 0.5g | **Carbohydrates:** 0.6g | **Fiber:** 0.3g

Grainy Mustard

A grainy mustard with some kick. Looking to make it hotter? Add more brown or black mustard seeds. Another option, add a little white wine to make it similar to a Dijon-style mustard, though this will add a few carbs.

Makes: 1 cup | **Serving Size:** 1 teaspoon

¼ cup yellow mustard seeds

¼ cup brown or black mustard seeds

¼ cup apple cider vinegar

¾ cup filtered water

¾ teaspoon salt

2½ teaspoons brown Swerve

1 tablespoon water

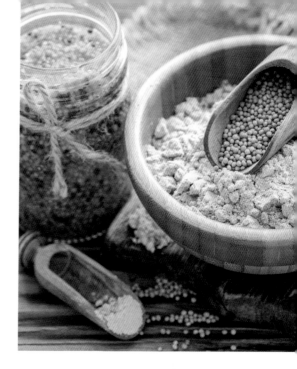

1. Add the mustard seeds, vinegar, and water to a jar with lid. Place in a cool, dark place for 24 to 48 hours to soak.

2. After the preferred time has elapsed, you'll notice the mustard seeds have settled to the bottom of the jar. Stir up the seeds to disburse evenly and then remove 1 tablespoon of seeds, including the liquid, and set aside.

3. Transfer the rest of the seeds and liquid to a blender along with the salt, Swerve, and water, and blend. If the mix is thicker than preferred, add another tablespoon of water.

4. When the desired consistency is reached, transfer the mixture to a container with a lid.

5. Stir in the reserved seeds and liquid.

6. Cover and refrigerate for 2 to 3 days for the flavor to develop before using. The longer the better.

7. Store in the fridge for up to a month in a glass jar.

NUTRITION PER SERVING: **Calories:** 2 | **Net Carbohydrates:** 0g | **Fat:** 0g | **Protein:** 0g | **Carbohydrates:** 0.1g | **Fiber:** 0.1g

Mustard Sauce

This sauce is inspired by the mustard-based sauces from the Carolinas. It's simply fabulous on a pork shoulder, pork ribs, and chicken. Baste it right on while grilling!

Makes: 1½ cups | **Serving Size:** 1 tablespoon

1 cup prepared Yellow Mustard (page 66)

2 tablespoons apple cider vinegar

2 teaspoons sea salt

½ teaspoon ground cayenne pepper

¼ cup brown Swerve

¾ teaspoon ground cloves

2 teaspoons Worcestershire sauce

¼ teaspoon cracked black peppercorns

½ teaspoon cayenne pepper hot sauce

1. Whisk all of the ingredients together in a small bowl and let sit for about 30 minutes before using.

2. Store sauce in a glass jar in the fridge for up to 2 weeks.

NUTRITION PER SERVING: **Calories:** 7 | **Net Carbohydrates:** 0.3g | **Fat:** 0.4g | **Protein:** 0.4g | **Carbohydrates:** 0.8g | **Fiber:** 0.5g

Soy Calamansi Sauce

This Filipino sauce is simple and tasty. Drizzle a little on some grilled chicken or fish.

Makes: ½ cup | **Serving Size:** 1 teaspoon

½ cup liquid aminos

1 tablespoon calamansi lime juice or key lime juice

1 bird's-eye chili, cut into rings

1. Whisk all of the ingredients together in a small bowl.

2. It's ready to be used immediately. Make as needed.

NUTRITION PER SERVING: **Calories:** 4 | **Net Carbohydrates:** 0.3g | **Fat:** 0g | **Protein:** 0.6g | **Carbohydrates:** 0.4g | **Fiber:** 0.1g

Gord's Blueberry Barbecue Sauce

I've known Jane and her husband Gord for years. When I ran into them during the summer, I shared this cookbook idea and Gord mentioned this blueberry barbecue sauce. It sounded intriguing. The original recipe's carb content was too high to be keto friendly, so I modified it somewhat using his recipe as inspiration. I never thought to use berries in a barbecue sauce, which then had me want to create a few more recipes with berries. This fruity barbecue sauce is fantastic with ribs and chicken. Slather it on while grilling.

Makes: 1½ cups | **Serving Size:** 2 tablespoons

1 tablespoon avocado oil

½ cup diced onions

3 cloves garlic, crushed

2 cups fresh blueberries

1 tablespoon granular Swerve

1 tablespoon brown Swerve

1 teaspoon Dijon mustard

½ teaspoon ground cumin

½ teaspoon smoked paprika

½ teaspoon ground chipotle chili

¼ teaspoon black pepper

2 teaspoons ancho chili powder

2 tablespoons apple cider vinegar

2 teaspoons Worcestershire sauce

½ teaspoon salt

1. Heat the avocado oil in a small saucepan over medium heat.

2. Add the onions and sauté for 2 to 3 minutes, until translucent.

3. Add the garlic and sauté for about 30 seconds, until fragrant.

4. Add the rest of the ingredients to the saucepan and bring to a boil.

5. Lower heat to a simmer and stir for 10 to 12 minutes, until the blueberries are broken down.

6. Blend with a stick blender to break down chunks until smooth.

7. Store in the fridge in a glass jar for up to 2 weeks.

NUTRITION PER SERVING: Calories: 35 | **Net Carbohydrates:** 4.5g | **Fat:** 1.5g | **Protein:** 0.4g | **Carbohydrates:** 5.5g | **Fiber:** 1g

Strawberry Basil Barbecue Sauce

This fruity, savory sauce is more like a glaze than a sauce. Glaze pork ribs or chicken 5 to 7 minutes before pulling them off the grill.

Makes: ¾ cup | **Serving Size:** 2 teaspoons

1 tablespoon avocado or olive oil

¼ cup diced onions

1 clove garlic, crushed

1 cup diced fresh strawberries

¼ cup chopped fresh basil

2 teaspoons Worcestershire sauce

2 tablespoons balsamic vinegar

1 teaspoon granular Swerve

¾ teaspoon sea salt

1. Heat the oil in a small saucepan over medium heat.

2. Once the oil is hot, add the onions and sauté for 2 to 3 minutes, until translucent.

3. Add the garlic and sauté for about 15 seconds, until fragrant.

4. Stir in the remaining ingredients.

5. Turn the heat down to low and simmer for 10 to 15 minutes, stirring occasionally to break down the strawberries.

6. After 15 minutes, turn off the heat and let cool.

7. Blend fine in a blender.

8. Store in a covered glass jar in the fridge for up to 2 weeks.

NUTRITION PER SERVING: **Calories:** 12 | **Net Carbohydrates:** 0.9g | **Fat:** 0.8g | **Protein:** 0.1g | **Carbohydrates:** 1.1g | **Fiber:** 0.2g

Cranberry Barbecue Sauce

While this sauce is cooking, the wafting scent may remind you of the holidays. You might be thinking turkey, but you'll want to slather this savory, herbaceous, slightly tart barbecue sauce on everything from beef and lamb to chicken and, yes, the occasional turkey.

Makes: 1 cup | **Serving Size:** 1 tablespoon

1 tablespoon avocado oil

½ medium onion, chopped

1 cup cranberries, fresh or frozen

½ tablespoon lemon juice

1 teaspoon apple cider vinegar

1 teaspoon Worcestershire sauce

1½ tablespoons brown Swerve

½ teaspoon dried thyme

½ teaspoon crushed dried rosemary

¼ teaspoon dried dill

½ tablespoon dried parsley

½ teaspoon sea salt

¼ teaspoon black pepper

6 tablespoons water

1. Heat the avocado oil in a saucepan over medium heat.

2. Add the onion and sauté for 2 minutes or until soft and translucent.

3. Stir in the remaining ingredients.

4. Reduce the heat to medium low and let the sauce cook, stirring occasionally.

5. Cook for about 10 to 15 minutes or until all the berries are broken down. If the sauce is becoming too thick, add additional water as needed, a tablespoon at a time.

6. Turn off the heat and blend the sauce smooth with a stick blender.

7. Transfer to a covered glass jar or container and refrigerate for up to 2 weeks.

NUTRITION PER SERVING: Calories: 14 | **Net Carbohydrates:** 1.2g | **Fat:** 0.9g | **Protein:** 0.1g | **Carbohydrates:** 1.6g | **Fiber:** 0.4g

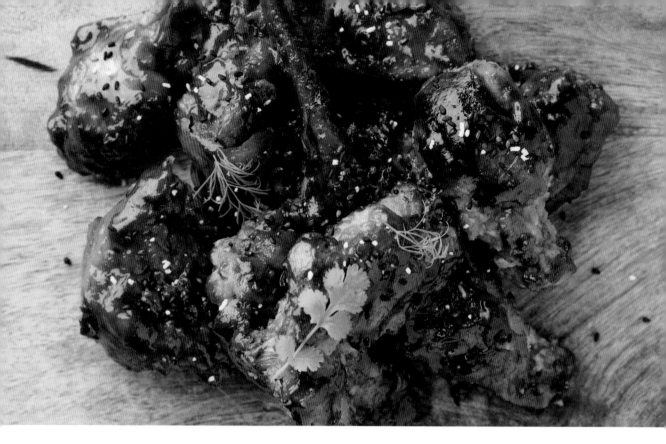

Korean Barbecue Sauce

Use about a third of this sauce to marinate dark chicken meat, then use about another third to baste while cooking. Sprinkle in a little xanthan gum to thicken the rest, and serve it at the table.

Makes: 2 cups | **Serving Size:** 1 tablespoon

1 cup liquid aminos

¾ cup brown Swerve

¾ teaspoon sesame oil

1 clove garlic, crushed

1 tablespoon rice vinegar

1 teaspoon chili paste or dried Korean chili flakes

1 teaspoon grated fresh ginger

½ teaspoon black pepper

⅛ teaspoon xanthan gum (optional)

1. Add all of the ingredients to a small saucepan over medium-low heat and heat for about 5 minutes. Stir occasionally to dissolve the sweetener.

2. Let cool before using.

3. Store in a covered glass jar in the fridge for up to 2 weeks.

NUTRITION PER SERVING: **Calories:** 7 | **Net Carbohydrates:** 0.5g | **Fat:** 0.1g | **Protein:** 1g | **Carbohydrates:** 0.6g | **Fiber:** 0.1g

Satay Sauce

A salty, savory peanut sauce. Serve it alongside grilled, chicken, pork, or beef strips.

Makes: ½ cup | **Serving Size:** 1 tablespoon

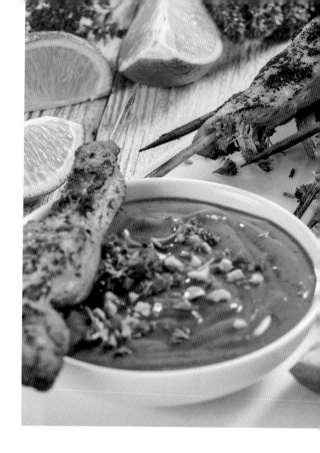

1 tablespoon avocado oil

1 clove garlic, crushed

½ tablespoon grated ginger

2 teaspoons liquid aminos

2 teaspoons lime juice

1 teaspoon fish sauce

2 tablespoons natural salted peanut butter

1 teaspoon chili paste or red pepper flakes

1 teaspoon brown Swerve

2 tablespoons water

1. Heat the avocado oil in a small saucepan over medium–low heat.

2. Once the oil is warm, add the garlic and ginger and gently sauté until fragrant, about 30 seconds.

3. Stir in the liquid aminos, lime juice, and fish sauce.

4. Next, whisk in the peanut butter, chili paste, and Swerve.

5. Once all of the ingredients are combined, slowly whisk in the water until desired consistency is reached.

6. Remove from heat, it's best served warm.

7. Store in the fridge in a covered glass jar for up to 2 weeks. Warm the sauce on the stove or in the microwave before using.

NUTRITION PER SERVING: Calories: 42 | **Net Carbohydrates:** 1.1g | **Fat:** 3.9g | **Protein:** 1.1g | **Carbohydrates:** 1.4g | **Fiber:** 0.3g

CHAPTER 5
Vinegar Sauces

Vinegar sauces are light, bright, tangy, and packed with flavor. You don't need a lot for impact as a little goes a long way.

Vinegar sauces pair great with fatty cuts of meat such as a pork shoulder or pork belly. The light, fresh acidity from the sauce adds a little balance to the heavier fatty cuts.

Store in the fridge in a glass jar (avoid storing in a metal container due to the high acidity) and use within a couple of weeks.

Carolina Vinegar Sauce

Drizzle this tangy sauce over pulled pork or serve on the side of pork belly burnt ends.

Makes: 1 cup | **Serving Size:** 1 tablespoon

1 cup apple cider vinegar

1 tablespoon brown Swerve

1 tablespoon sugar–free ketchup

½ teaspoon sea salt

1. Whisk all of the ingredients together in a small bowl and infuse in the fridge overnight.

2. Store in a glass jar with a lid for up to 2 weeks.

NUTRITION PER SERVING: **Calories:** 3 | **Net Carbohydrates:** 0.2g |
Fat: 0g | **Protein:** 0g | **Carbohydrates:** 0.2g | **Fiber:** 0g

Garlic Vinegar Sauce

Another one of my childhood favorites. The garlic flavor infuses into the vinegar, creating a sauce that goes great with greasier foods. Try it with fattier cuts of beef or pork.

Makes: ½ cup | **Serving Size:** 1 teaspoon

½ cup white vinegar

1 clove garlic, crushed

¼ teaspoon salt

⅛ teaspoon cracked black peppercorns

pinch of confectioner's Swerve (optional)

1 bird's-eye chili, cut into rings

1. Whisk all of the ingredients together in a small bowl and infuse for 15 to 20 minutes.

2. This sauce is best when made and eaten as needed.

NUTRITION PER SERVING: Calories: 2 | **Net Carbohydrates:** 0.2g | **Fat:** 0g | **Protein:** 0g | **Carbohydrates:** 0.2g | **Fiber:** 0g

Mop Sauce

Use this sauce to keep turkey, pork shoulder, and beef ribs moist while in the smoker. Reserve about a third of a cup to enjoy with that pulled pork.

Makes: 1¼ cups | **Serving Size:** 1 tablespoon

1 cup filtered water

2 tablespoons sugar-free ketchup

1½ tablespoons apple cider vinegar

1 teaspoon white vinegar

⅛ teaspoon ground cayenne pepper

⅛ teaspoon black pepper

⅛ teaspoon sea salt

½ teaspoon brown Swerve

1. Whisk all of the ingredients together in a medium bowl.

2. Use with a basting brush or a sauce mop.

3. Discard used mop sauce.

NUTRITION PER SERVING: Calories: 1 | **Net Carbohydrates:** 0.1g | **Fat:** 0g | **Protein:** 0g | **Carbohydrates:** 0.1g | **Fiber:** 0g

Savory Spritz

Use this savory spritz to keep those large proteins like beef ribs and brisket moist in the smoker. Adds a touch of flavor and lots of moisture for those long cooks.

Makes: 1 cup | **Serving Size:** 1 teaspoon

1 cup filtered water

2 tablespoons apple cider vinegar

1 tablespoon Worcestershire sauce

2 teaspoons sugar-free ketchup

1. Add the water, vinegar, and Worcestershire sauce to a small bowl and mix.

2. Whisk in the ketchup.

3. Transfer to a food-safe spray bottle.

4. Discard any leftovers.

NUTRITION PER SERVING: **Calories:** 0 | **Net Carbohydrates:** 0.1g | **Fat:** 0g | **Protein:** 0g | **Carbohydrates:** 0.1g | **Fiber:** 0g

CHAPTER 6

Mayonnaises and Aioli

Mayonnaise is an emulsion (a mixture) of two components, oil and water, that don't typically mix or stay mixed on their own. To help this process, usually a whole egg or an egg yolk brings the oil and water together to form a fatty, delicious, creamy condiment. It can be a tricky process where at any point, this mixture can "break" and separate, leaving an undesirable oily layer on top. In that case, certain tricks can fix the emulsion, but they don't always work.

This fatty condiment can supplement the higher fat intake that is required by the keto diet, and it's especially convenient when you can make it yourself and choose the ingredients.

Store-bought mayonnaise usually contains sugar, canola, or soybean oil along with emulsifiers to keep the mayonnaise from separating while on the shelf.

In a pinch commercial mayonnaise is convenient to use but once you learn how to make it with ingredients you choose, you may never go back to store-bought mayonnaise again.

Components

"EGG": Normally, a whole egg or egg yolk is used to help emulsification. If you're a little uneasy with using raw eggs, consider using carton eggs or egg yolks, which are pasteurized. There are other egglike alternatives that work too, like flax.

ACID: The liquid component that adds flavor. Usually it's white vinegar along with a little lemon juice, which imparts a freshness. Try using a different vinegar to change things up. Normally 2 tablespoons of acid are needed.

MUSTARD: Mustard can also aid in the emulsification process. Dried or prepared yellow mustard or even Dijon mustard work while adding flavor. Usually ½ to 1 teaspoon is needed.

OIL: A neutral oil such as avocado or a light olive oil fares well, especially when using the mayonnaise in other recipes. That being said, oils/fats with more flavor, like nut oils or melted bacon fat, can also work. They'll just have a unique flavor. Use oils alone or in combination to create a blend—it's fun to experiment!

SEASONINGS: Salt is a must. In regular mayonnaise, the flavors come from their individual components and salt just amplifies them. You're definitely not limited to salt alone. Try using different flavored salts. Herbs and spices add another twist. Just add them after the mayonnaise has been made.

Aioli

The traditional aioli originated in the Mediterranean and is also an emulsion. Its components are also incredibly simple yet difficult to prepare. Aioli translated from French is just garlic (*ai*) and oil (*oli*). Made in the traditional way with the use of a mortar and pestle, it consists of fresh garlic, extra-virgin olive oil, and salt. Crush the garlic cloves in the mortar along with a little salt to add abrasiveness. Then, once the garlic is well crushed, slowly drizzle in the olive oil while continuing to crush the garlic. This gradually emulsifies the garlic and oil but needs to be done continuously to avoid breaking the emulsion. You can achieve a paste-like consistency after a minute or so. I've tried working in more olive oil, hoping to achieve that creamy consistency beyond the garlic paste, but the emulsion "broke" and I was left with an oily mess! It's a task for another day. A traditional aioli requires a little more garlic, which is higher in carbs.

More modern methods use an egg to help with emulsification and a food processor to make the task easier.

Nowadays, an "aioli" refers to a garlic-flavored mayonnaise but it's also become synonymous for all flavored mayonnaises.

In cooking, mayonnaises and aiolis are a perfect combination. That little bit of protein from the egg along with the added oil will add another dimension of flavor.

Uses

CONDIMENT: Serve on burgers, slather on top of meats and grilled vegetables, use as a dip for just about everything.

MARINADE: Mix in more acid and flavorings for use as a marinade.

COOKING: Already chock-full of flavorful fats, use it to baste proteins on the grill to keep them moist.

Stick Blender Mayonnaise

Bypassing the need to continuously drizzle oil, this method to make mayonnaise is a little easier. The whole process takes place in one jar that you can then use to cover and store the mayonnaise. This particular recipe uses an extra egg; it's not necessary but I find it helpful.

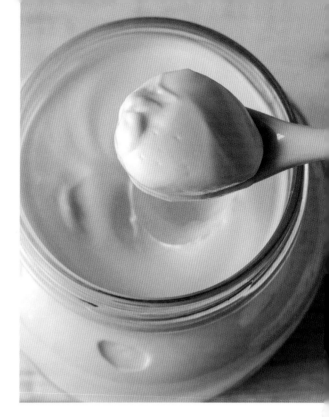

Makes: 1¼ cups | **Serving Size:** 1 tablespoon

1 tablespoon white vinegar

1 tablespoon lemon juice (optional)

½ teaspoon salt

½ teaspoon mustard powder

2 eggs

1 cup avocado oil or extra-virgin olive oil

pinch of granular Swerve

1. To a 1.5-pint, wide-mouth canning jar, add the vinegar, lemon juice (if desired), salt, mustard powder, and eggs.

2. Next, pour the oil carefully so it sits on top.

3. Place a stick blender all the way to the bottom of the jar and turn on Blend until the ingredients at the bottom of the jar are emulsified.

4. Then, while blending, bring the blender about a quarter of the way up, and hold it in place.

5. Once the oil is emulsified, slowly raise the blender halfway or three quarter of the way to incorporate the remaining oil.

6. Cover and store in the fridge for up to a week.

NUTRITION PER SERVING: Calories: 104 | **Net Carbohydrates:** 0.1g | **Fat:** 11.4g | **Protein:** 0.6g | **Carbohydrates:** 0.1g | **Fiber:** 0g

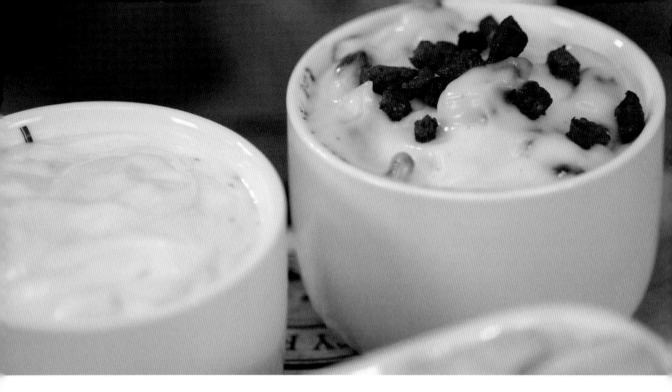

Bacon Mayonnaise

What's better for keto and barbecues than bacon mayonnaise?
It's a delicious way to get those fats in with a burger.

Makes: 1 cup | **Serving Size:** 1 tablespoon

1 egg yolk

½ teaspoon smoked sea salt

½ tablespoon apple cider vinegar

½ tablespoon white vinegar

½ teaspoon mushroom powder

1 tablespoon avocado oil

1 cup bacon fat, melted and cooled

½ teaspoon smoked paprika

pinch of granular or confectioner's Swerve

1. Add the egg yolk, salt, vinegars, and mushroom powder to a food processor and blend.

2. Slowly drizzle in a steady stream of the avocado oil followed by the bacon fat while whisking or blending, occasionally pausing to ensure that the fat is incorporated fully.

3. Once the fats have been emulsified, whisk in the paprika and Swerve.

4. Transfer the mayonnaise to an airtight container and store in the fridge for up to a week.

NUTRITION PER SERVING: Calories: 128 | **Net Carbohydrates:** 0.2g |
Fat: 14g | **Protein:** 0.2g | **Carbohydrates:** 0.2g | **Fiber:** 0g

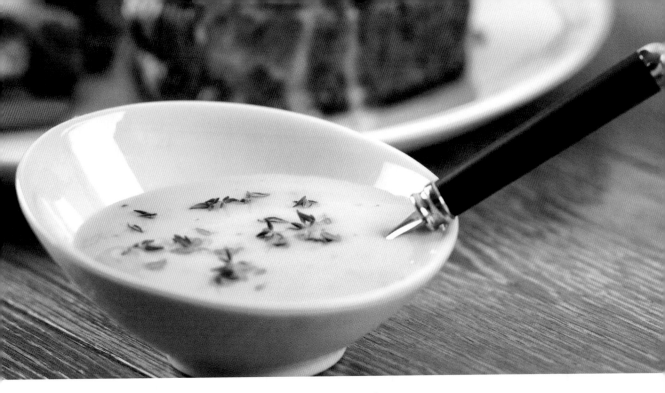

Bearnaise

This velvety, buttery, emulsified sauce makes steak all the more mouthwatering. It's best when it's fresh and used soon after making, as it may harden when refrigerated. If refrigerated, just let it come to room temperature and give it a stir before serving.

Makes: 1 cup | **Serving Size:** 1 tablespoon

2 egg yolks

¼ teaspoon sea salt

2 tablespoons lemon juice

1 cup melted butter/ghee, cooled

1½ tablespoons chopped fresh parsley

1½ tablespoons chopped scallions or chives

1. In a food processor, blend the egg yolks, salt, and lemon juice.

2. Once the sauce is well blended, keep the food processor blending and slowly drizzle in the melted butter.

3. After the butter has emulsified completely, stir in the parsley and scallions.

4. Transfer to a small bowl.

5. This sauce is best when made fresh.

NUTRITION PER SERVING: Calories: 109 | **Net Carbohydrates:** 0.3g | **Fat:** 12.1g | **Protein:** 0.5g | **Carbohydrates:** 0.3g | **Fiber:** 0g

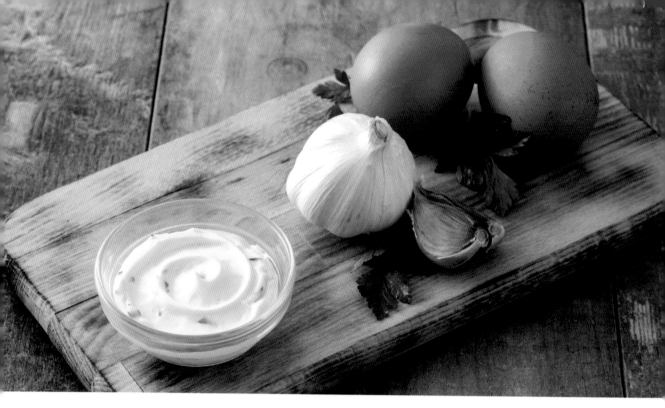

Aioli

As mentioned previously, a traditional aioli is just garlic and olive oil but tricky to make. This method uses power tools and an egg to help with emulsification. It's rich and creamy with that garlic kick.

Makes: 1¼ cups | **Serving Size:** 1 tablespoon

2 cloves garlic, roughly chopped

¼ teaspoon mustard powder

1 tablespoon lemon juice

1 tablespoon white vinegar

½ teaspoon salt

1 egg yolk

1 cup extra-virgin olive oil

1. In a food processor with a 2-cup capacity, blend the garlic, mustard powder, lemon juice, white vinegar, salt, and egg yolk.

2. While the food processor is still running, slowly drizzle in the olive oil through the access spout. Make sure the oil is being incorporated. If it looks like it's pooling on top, stop drizzling and wait until the oil gone. Once the oil on top is has emulsified, continue adding the rest of the oil.

3. Transfer the aioli to a jar and store in the fridge for up to a week.

NUTRITION PER SERVING: **Calories:** 103 | **Net Carbohydrates:** 0.2g | **Fat:** 11.7g | **Protein:** 0.5g | **Carbohydrates:** 0.2g | **Fiber:** 0g

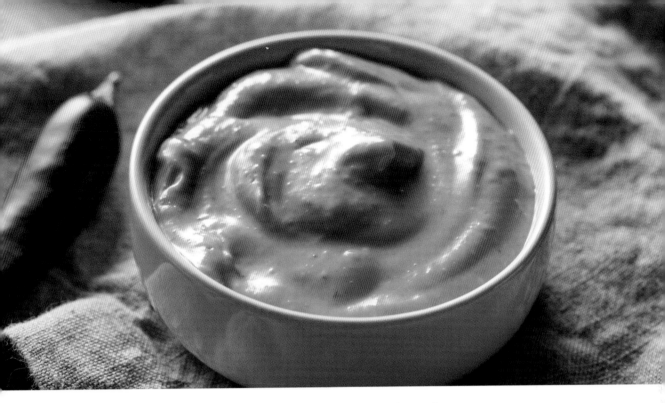

Chipotle Aioli

A good raw or grilled vegetable dip or baste for chicken thighs on the grill.

Makes: 1 cup | **Serving Size:** 1 tablespoon

1 cup mayonnaise

¼ teaspoon chipotle chili powder

½ teaspoon smoked paprika

⅛ teaspoon garlic powder

¼ teaspoon sea salt

1. Whisk all of the ingredients together in a small bowl.

2. Infuse in the fridge for at least an hour, before using for the flavors to mix.

3. Store in the fridge in a glass jar or in a ready-to-use squeezable plastic condiment bottle. Use within a week.

NUTRITION PER SERVING: **Calories:** 94 | **Net Carbohydrates:** 0.2g | **Fat:** 10.3g | **Protein:** 0.2g | **Carbohydrates:** 0.2g | **Fiber:** 0g

Maple Mustard Aioli

A slightly different version from sweet mustard, this maple mustard aioli uses maple instead of honey. It goes well with that smoky pulled pork or as a dip for grilled chicken.

Makes: ¾ cup | **Serving Size:** 1 tablespoon

2 teaspoons apple cider vinegar

½ teaspoon maple extract

1½ tablespoons brown Swerve

2 tablespoons Grainy Mustard (page 67) or Dijon mustard or ¼ cup Yellow Mustard (page 66)

½ cup mayonnaise

1. Whisk the vinegar, maple extract, and Swerve together in a small bowl. Let sit for 10 minutes or so for the sweetener to dissolve.

2. Mix the mustard and mayonnaise together in a separate bowl, then whisk in the vinegar solution.

3. Cover and place the aioli in the fridge for an hour or so to let the flavors mix.

4. Stir well before serving.

5. Store in the fridge in a covered glass or plastic container for up to a week.

NUTRITION PER SERVING: Calories: 66 | **Net Carbohydrates:** 0.1g | **Fat:** 6.9g | **Protein:** 0.1g | **Carbohydrates:** 0.1g | **Fiber:** 0g

Mustard Aioli

Good on bratwurst, smokies, or beef.

Makes: ¾ cup | **Serving Size:** 1 tablespoon

½ cup Yellow Mustard (page 66) or Grainy Mustard (page 67)

½ cup mayonnaise

½ teaspoon dried thyme

½ teaspoon paprika

½ teaspoon Swerve

2 teaspoons finely chopped fresh flat leaf parsley

1 tablespoon scallion, chopped

½ teaspoon sea salt

1. Whisk all of the ingredients together in a medium bowl.

2. Cover and infuse in the fridge for at least an hour before using.

3. Store in the fridge in a glass jar or a plastic condiment squeeze bottle for up to a week.

NUTRITION PER SERVING: Calories: 69 | **Net Carbohydrates:** 0.3g | **Fat:** 7.2g | **Protein:** 0.5g | **Carbohydrates:** 0.8g | **Fiber:** 0.5g

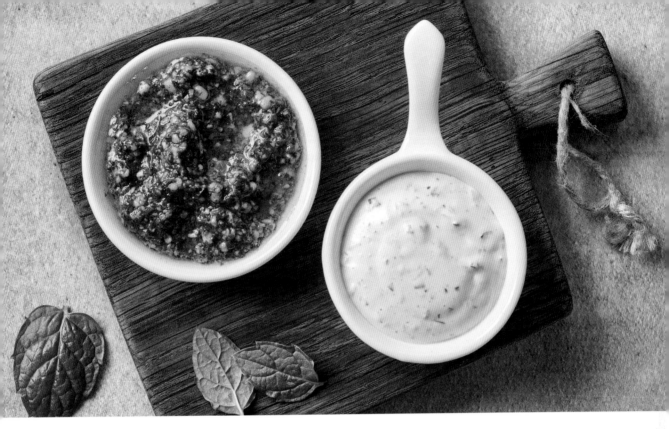

Pesto Aioli

A creamy, garlicky, savory aioli to spread on chicken breasts and fish before grilling.

Makes: ¾ cup | **Serving Size:** 1 tablespoon

¼ cup Basic Pesto (page 110)

½ cup mayonnaise

1 tablespoon lemon juice

¼ teaspoon granular or confectioner's Swerve

¼ teaspoon sea salt

1. Whisk all of the ingredients together in a medium bowl.

2. Cover and infuse in the fridge for 15 minutes before using.

3. Store in the fridge in a covered glass container and use within a week.

NUTRITION PER SERVING: **Calories:** 106 | **Net Carbohydrates:** 0.8g | **Fat:** 11g | **Protein:** 0.9g | **Carbohydrates:** 1g | **Fiber:** 0.2g

Sriracha Aioli

A must-try on pulled pork. Or, drizzle on smoked chicken. If you'd like the sauce to be a thicker, use a little bit of xanthan gum.

Makes: 1¼ cups | **Serving Size:** 1 tablespoon

1 cup mayonnaise

¼ cup sriracha

2 teaspoons brown Swerve

2 tablespoons lime juice

½ teaspoon garlic powder

¾ teaspoon salt

1. Whisk all of the ingredients together in a medium bowl.

2. Cover and infuse in the fridge for at least an hour before using.

3. Store in the fridge in a covered glass jar for up to a week.

> **NUTRITION PER SERVING: Calories:** 78 | **Net Carbohydrates:** 0.8g | **Fat:** 8.3g | **Protein:** 0.2g | **Carbohydrates:** 0.9g | **Fiber:** 0.1g

Wasabi Aioli

A rich, savory aioli. Use it as a condiment to serve with grilled salmon, or slather it on top of fish before grilling.

Makes: ½ cup | **Serving Size:** 1 tablespoon

½ cup mayonnaise

2 teaspoons wasabi

1 tablespoon liquid aminos

pinch of granular or confectioner's Swerve

⅛ teaspoon powdered ginger or ginger juice (optional)

1. Whisk all of the ingredients together in a small bowl.

2. Infuse in the fridge for at least an hour before using.

3. Store in the fridge for up to a week.

> **NUTRITION PER SERVING: Calories:** 98 | **Net Carbohydrates:** 0.7g | **Fat:** 10.5g | **Protein:** 0.2g | **Carbohydrates:** 0.8g | **Fiber:** 0.1g

CHAPTER 7
Dips and Dressings

I'm a little obsessed with dips and love dipping things in dips! From raw cut vegetables to wings, riblets, and grilled chicken, there's nothing as satisfying as dunking and enrobing them in a creamy, tangy, and tasty dip.

The next time you're invited to a potluck barbecue, bring a few of these dips along with a platter of raw cut vegetables (broccoli, bell pepper strips, cauliflower, cucumber, and zucchini are great keto-friendly vegetables). Everyone will want to try all the dips and discover their new favorite.

If the sour cream is a little too rich, substitute full-fat yogurt. Just keep in mind that it may add a few more carbs, depending on the yogurt you use.

With the variety of flavors, you'll want to try using it in other ways:

- Thin out the dip with a little bit of almond milk or water and use as a salad dressing or a marinade.

- Thin out the dip with a little bit of heavy cream, place it in a condiment squeeze bottle, and drizzle it on top of grilled foods.

- Use it as is on top of your favorite burger.

- Use it as a side with barbecued or grilled meats.

- Baste it on as is while grilling.

Store the dips and dressings in the fridge up to the sour cream expiration date.

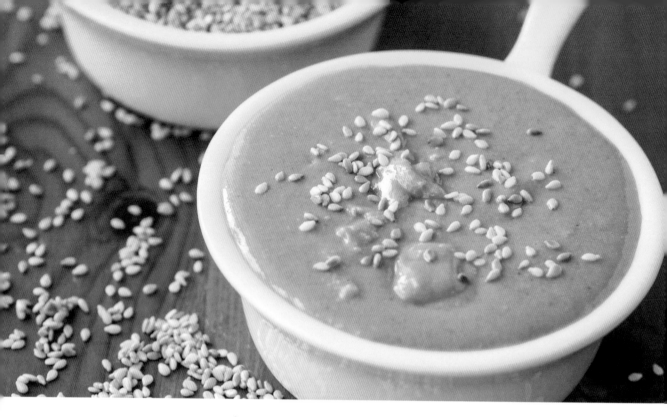

Asian Sesame Dip

A nice flavorful sauce for dipping. Thin it out a little with water or unsweetened almond milk and toss with grated cabbage and roasted sesame seeds for an Asian-inspired slaw.

Makes: 1 cup | **Serving Size:** 1 tablespoon

½ cup mayonnaise

½ cup full-fat sour cream

3 tablespoons liquid aminos

1½ tablespoons rice vinegar

1½ teaspoons sesame oil

½ teaspoon garlic powder

½ teaspoon onion powder

1. Whisk all of the ingredients together in a medium bowl.

2. Cover and infuse in the fridge for a few hours before using.

3. Store in the fridge in a covered glass or plastic container up to the sour cream expiration date.

NUTRITION PER SERVING: Calories: 62 | **Net Carbohydrates:** 0.5g | **Fat:** 6.6g | **Protein:** 0.3g | **Carbohydrates:** 0.5g | **Fiber:** 0g

Blue Cheese Buffalo Dip

A mild rich and cheesy dip with a hint of buffalo for everyone to enjoy. Add more hot sauce if you like it hotter, then dip some grilled wings or grilled cauliflower in.

Makes: 1½ cups | **Serving Size:** 1 tablespoon

¼ cup cream cheese

2 tablespoons salted butter

½ cup mayonnaise

½ cup full-fat sour cream

2 tablespoons crumbled blue cheese

1½ tablespoons cayenne pepper hot sauce

¾ teaspoon sea salt

1. Place the cream cheese and butter in a small microwave-safe bowl. Melt in the microwave for about 30 seconds.

2. Mix the rest of the ingredients together in a separate bowl, then whisk in the melted cream cheese and butter, and the dip is ready to use.

3. Store in the fridge in a covered glass or plastic container up to the sour cream or cheese expiration date, whichever comes first.

NUTRITION PER SERVING: **Calories:** 62 | **Net Carbohydrates:** 0.4g | **Fat:** 6.5g | **Protein:** 0.6g | **Carbohydrates:** 0.4g | **Fiber:** 0g

Chili Lime Dip

Smoky, tangy, and incredibly savory. A bold sauce to bring out the best in seafood and fish. One of my favorites!

Makes: 1 cup | **Serving Size:** 1 tablespoon

½ cup mayonnaise

½ cup full–fat sour cream

½ teaspoon chipotle chili pepper powder

2 tablespoons lime juice

2 teaspoons ancho chili powder

½ teaspoon granular or confectioner's Swerve

2 teaspoons lime zest

¾ teaspoon citric acid

1 teaspoon sea salt

1. Whisk all of the ingredients together in a medium bowl.

2. Cover and infuse in the fridge for a few hours before using.

3. Store in the fridge in a covered glass or plastic container up to the sour cream expiration date.

NUTRITION PER SERVING: **Calories:** 62 | **Net Carbohydrates:** 0.6g | **Fat:** 6.6g | **Protein:** 0.3g | **Carbohydrates:** 0.8g | **Fiber:** 0.2g

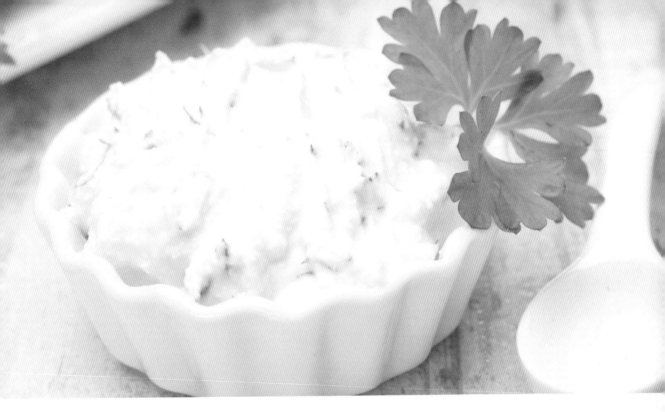

Greek Feta Dip

Serve this with grilled chicken skewers or thin it out a little with water or unsweetened almond milk for a creamy Greek salad dressing.

Makes: 1¼ cups | **Serving Size:** 1 tablespoon

½ cup mayonnaise

½ cup full-fat sour cream

¼ cup crumbled feta

2 teaspoons dried dill

1 teaspoon dried thyme

1 teaspoon dried oregano

½ teaspoon sea salt

½ teaspoon granulated or confectioner's Swerve

2 turns coarse black peppercorns

1. Whisk all of the ingredients together in a medium bowl.

2. Cover and infuse in the fridge for a few hours before using.

3. Store in the fridge in a covered glass or plastic container up to the sour cream or cheese expiration date, whichever comes first.

NUTRITION PER SERVING: Calories: 54 | **Net Carbohydrates:** 0.5g | **Fat:** 5.6g | **Protein:** 0.5g | **Carbohydrates:** 0.6g | **Fiber:** 0.1g

Roasted Garlic, Parmesan, and Chives Dip

Marvelous for dipping cut veggies. Try tossing some grilled shrimp into this dip and add to a Caesar salad.

Makes: about 1⅓ cups | **Serving Size:** 2 tablespoons

½ cup mayonnaise

½ cup full-fat sour cream

1 tablespoon finely chopped fresh chives

4 cloves roasted minced garlic

3 tablespoons powdered Parmesan cheese

½ teaspoon sea salt

¼ teaspoon black pepper

1. Mix the mayonnaise and sour cream in a small bowl.

2. Stir in the remaining ingredients.

3. Cover and place in the fridge for a few hours before using, for the flavors to develop.

4. Store in the fridge in a covered glass or plastic container up to the sour cream or cheese expiration date, whichever comes first.

NUTRITION PER SERVING: Calories: 102 | **Net Carbohydrates:** 1.2g | **Fat:** 10.3g | **Protein:** 1.3g | **Carbohydrates:** 1.2g | **Fiber:** 0g

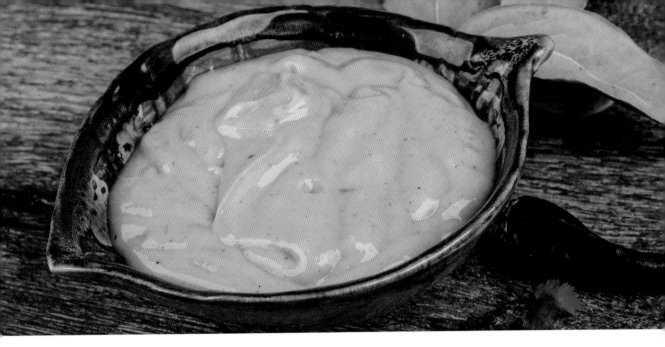

Yellow Curry Dip

A mild curry for dipping vegetables or marinating chicken or fish. If you like it spicier, just increase the amount of cayenne powder.

Makes: 1 cup | **Serving Size:** 1 tablespoon

½ cup mayonnaise

½ cup full–fat sour cream

1 teaspoon ground turmeric

1 tablespoon ground cumin

1 tablespoon ground coriander

¼ teaspoon mustard powder

¼ teaspoon ground ginger

⅛ teaspoon ground cayenne pepper

½ teaspoon sea salt

1. Whisk all of the ingredients together in a small bowl.

2. Cover and place in the fridge for a few hours before using, for the flavors to develop.

3. Store in the fridge in a covered glass or plastic container up to the sour cream expiration date.

NUTRITION PER SERVING: **Calories:** 64 | **Net Carbohydrates:** 0.7g | **Fat:** 6.7g | **Protein:** 0.4g | **Carbohydrates:** 0.9g | **Fiber:** 0.2g

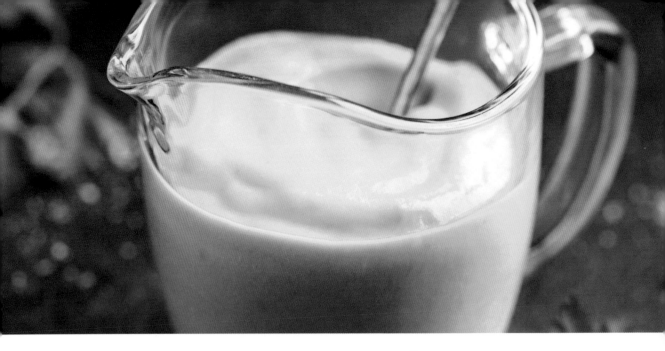

Avocado Dressing

This dressing has a slightly chunky texture. If you prefer a smooth texture throughout, blend all of the ingredients together. Toss this dressing in with a leafy green salad or drizzle it on grilled beef, pork, or chicken strips.

Makes: ½ cup | **Serving Size:** 2 tablespoons

½ avocado, chopped

¼ cup full-fat sour cream

½ teaspoon sea salt

¼ teaspoon ground cumin

¼ teaspoon cracked whole coriander

⅛ teaspoon citric acid

¼ teaspoon granular Swerve

1 tablespoon lime juice

¼ teaspoon smoked paprika

¼ teaspoon garlic powder

1 tablespoon chopped cilantro (optional)

½ teaspoon dried onion

½ avocado, mashed

1. Blend the ½ chopped avocado, sour cream, salt, cumin, coriander, citric acid, Swerve, lime juice, smoked paprika, garlic powder, and cilantro, if using, in a small bowl until smooth.

2. Mix in the dried onion and mashed avocado.

3. Cover and infuse in the fridge for at least 30 minutes before using.

4. Store in the fridge in a covered glass container for up to 2 days.

NUTRITION PER SERVING: **Calories:** 92 | **Net Carbohydrates:** 2.1g | **Fat:** 8.4g | **Protein:** 1.2g | **Carbohydrates:** 4.8g | **Fiber:** 2.7g

Ranch Dressing

Try basting this popular dressing on grilled foods while cooking.

Makes: 1¼ cups | **Serving Size:** 1 tablespoon

1 cup mayonnaise

¼ cup sour cream

1 teaspoon dried chives

1 teaspoon dried dill

1 teaspoon dried parsley

½ teaspoon garlic powder

½ teaspoon onion powder

1 teaspoon mustard powder

1 tablespoon lemon juice or buttermilk

½ teaspoon salt

¼ teaspoon black pepper

1. Whisk all of the ingredients together in a medium bowl.

2. Cover and infuse in the fridge for a few hours before using.

3. Store in the fridge in a covered glass or plastic container up to the sour cream or buttermilk (if used) expiration date, whichever comes first.

NUTRITION PER SERVING: Calories: 82 | **Net Carbohydrates:** 0.4g | **Fat:** 8.8g | **Protein:** 0.2g | **Carbohydrates:** 0.4g | **Fiber:** 0g

Smoky Caesar

Putting a little twist on the full-fat Caesar dressing, this recipe adds a little bit of smokiness that's perfect on chicken, beef, and salmon. It's also good with grilled zucchini and cauliflower.

Makes: 1 cup | **Serving Size:** 1 tablespoon

1 cup mayonnaise

2 teaspoons smoked paprika

1 tablespoon powdered Parmesan cheese

4 teaspoons lemon juice

1 teaspoon anchovy paste or Worcestershire sauce

1 teaspoon whole grain or Dijon mustard

1 teaspoon extra-virgin olive oil

2 cloves garlic, crushed

¼ teaspoon salt

¼ teaspoon coarse black peppercorns, cracked

1. Whisk all of the ingredients together in a medium bowl.

2. Cover and infuse in the fridge for a couple of hours before using.

3 Store in the fridge in a covered glass or plastic container up to 2 weeks.

NUTRITION PER SERVING: Calories: 105 | **Net Carbohydrates:** 0.4g | **Fat:** 11.3g | **Protein:** 0.4g | **Carbohydrates:** 0.5g | **Fiber:** 0.1g

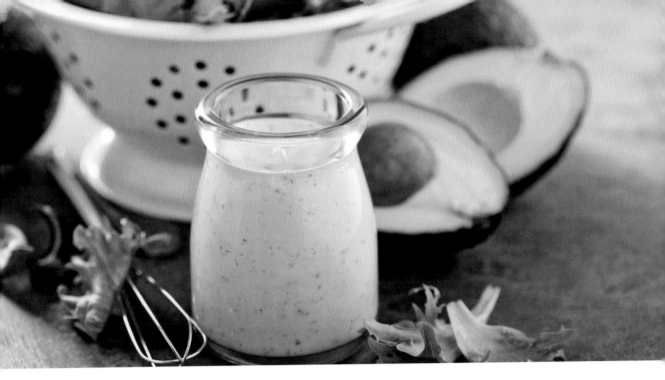

Green Goddess Dressing

This savory dressing is fantastic for drizzling on meats and use as a burger condiment. Dip chicken wings in it too!

Makes: 1¼ cups | **Serving Size:** 1 tablespoon

1 cup mayonnaise

2 tablespoons lemon juice

2 teaspoons Swerve

2 teaspoons chopped green onion

2 tablespoons chopped fresh basil

1 teaspoon anchovy paste

1 tablespoon chopped fresh parsley

1 tablespoon apple cider vinegar

¼ cup full-fat sour cream

1 tablespoon chopped tarragon

½ teaspoon onion powder

½ teaspoon citric acid

½ teaspoon sea salt

2 turns coarse black peppercorns

1. Mix all of the ingredients together in a medium bowl.

2. Cover and infuse in the fridge for a couple of hours before using.

3. Store in the fridge in a covered glass or plastic container up to the sour cream expiration date.

NUTRITION PER SERVING: Calories: 82 | **Net Carbohydrates:** 0.5g | **Fat:** 8.8g | **Protein:** 0.3g | **Carbohydrates:** 0.5g | **Fiber:** 0g

CHAPTER 8

Compound Butters

A compound butter is a butter with herbs and/or spices mixed in and then refrigerated.

Compound butters are convenient to have available, just slice some off what you need it. Store them in the fridge or longer term in the freezer. Have a few different flavors ready to go for that impromptu grilling session.

Uses for compound butters:

- Cooking: Melt down the butter in a heatproof dish on a cooler part of the barbecue, and use it for basting.
- Self-basting: Place a few tablespoons of the butter on top of chicken, fish, steak, or seafood at the start of cooking. While it cooks on the grill, the butter melts and disperses the seasonings.
- Finishing: When the steaks, fish, seafood, or veggies come off the grill (or just before), top with a tablespoon of compound butter.
- Serving: Keep a few pats of compound butter at the table.

Steps:

1. Use 1 stick (½ cup) of softened salted butter.

2. Choose one of the combinations in the recipes below, or come up with one of your own. Fresh herbs (such as basil, cilantro, chives, dill, parsley, rosemary, sage, and scallions) are great to use—they stay "fresh" in the butter.

3. Chop the herbs and mix them in with the salted butter.

4. Position a piece of plastic wrap or parchment paper, about the size of a piece of paper (8½ x 11 inches) in a landscape orientation, and spoon the compound butter mixture on it.

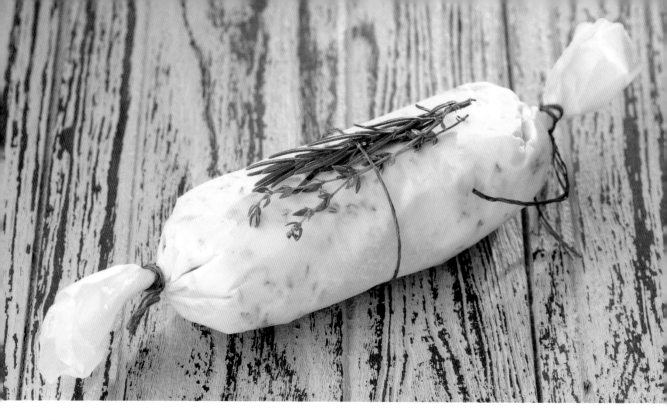

5. Carefully mold and roll the butter into a 4-inch log using the sides of the wrap or parchment. The diameter of the log will be about the size of a dollar coin.

6. Twist the ends of the plastic wrap or parchment paper and label it with the seasonings and the date.

7. Place in the fridge to harden or in the freezer for longer-term storage, up to 3 months.

8. When you're ready to use it, just unroll and slice off what you need. If you score it into 8 pieces, the portion size is approximately 1 tablespoon.

Compound Butters for Beef and Steak

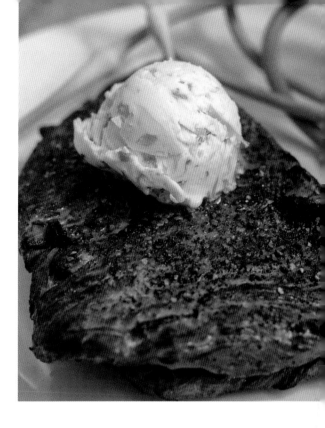

1 teaspoon dried thyme

1 teaspoon dried rosemary

2 cloves garlic, roasted

NUTRITION PER SERVING: Calories: 103 | **Net Carbohydrates:** 0.4g | **Fat:** 11.5g | **Protein:** 0.2g | **Carbohydrates:** 0.5g | **Fiber:** 0.1g

½ teaspoon chipotle chili pepper powder

1 teaspoon dried oregano

½ teaspoon ground cumin

NUTRITION PER SERVING: Calories: 103 | **Net Carbohydrates:** 0.1g | **Fat:** 11.5g | **Protein:** 0.2g | **Carbohydrates:** 0.3g | **Fiber:** 0.2g

Compound Butters for Chicken

1 sundried tomato, chopped

2 cloves garlic, roasted

2 teaspoons capers, drained

NUTRITION PER SERVING: Calories: 103 | **Net Carbohydrates:** 0.3g | **Fat:** 11.5g | **Protein:** 0.2g | **Carbohydrates:** 0.4g | **Fiber:** 0.1g

2 teaspoons dried dill

1 teaspoon dried thyme

NUTRITION PER SERVING: Calories: 102 | **Net Carbohydrates:** 0.2g | **Fat:** 11.5g | **Protein:** 0.2g | **Carbohydrates:** 0.3g | **Fiber:** 0.1g

1 tablespoon crumbled bacon

2 teaspoons chopped scallions

NUTRITION PER SERVING: Calories: 110 | **Net Carbohydrates:** 0.1g | **Fat:** 12.1g | **Protein:** 0.8g | **Carbohydrates:** 0.1g | **Fiber:** 0g

Compound Butters
for Fish and Seafood

1 sundried tomato, chopped

1½ teaspoons capers, drained

1 teaspoon dried dill

NUTRITION PER SERVING: **Calories:** 102 | **Net Carbohydrates:** 0.1g | **Fat:** 11.5g | **Protein:** 0.2g | **Carbohydrates:** 0.2g | **Fiber:** 0.1g

1 tablespoon roasted seaweed strips

1 teaspoon wasabi

1 teaspoon roasted sesame seeds

NUTRITION PER SERVING: **Calories:** 108 | **Net Carbohydrates:** 0.5g | **Fat:** 11.9g | **Protein:** 0.3g | **Carbohydrates:** 0.6g | **Fiber:** 0.1g

1 clove garlic, crushed

1 tablespoon finely chopped fresh parsley

1½ teaspoons fresh thyme

NUTRITION PER SERVING: **Calories:** 102 | **Net Carbohydrates:** 0.2g | **Fat:** 11.5g | **Protein:** 0.2g | **Carbohydrates:** 0.2g | **Fiber:** 0g

Compound Butters
for Grilled Vegetables

1½ tablespoons crumbled blue cheese

1 teaspoon dried thyme

1½ teaspoons dried oregano

NUTRITION PER SERVING: **Calories:** 107 | **Net Carbohydrates:** 0.2g | **Fat:** 11.9g | **Protein:** 0.5g | **Carbohydrates:** 0.3g | **Fiber:** 0.1g

1 teaspoon dried tarragon

1½ teaspoons horseradish

1½ teaspoons capers, drained

NUTRITION PER SERVING: **Calories:** 107 | **Net Carbohydrates:** 0.2g | **Fat:** 12.0g | **Protein:** 0.2g | **Carbohydrates:** 0.2g | **Fiber:** 0g

1½ tablespoons finely chopped scallions

2 cloves garlic, roasted

NUTRITION PER SERVING: **Calories:** 103 | **Net Carbohydrates:** 0.3g | **Fat:** 11.5g | **Protein:** 0.2g | **Carbohydrates:** 0.3g | **Fiber:** 0g

CHAPTER 9

Compound Sauces

I was a little unsure what to call this lovely group of sauces. I find that they're complex in flavor and use components with some dimension (e.g., chunky). Most require a little stirring to mix up before using. Some are incredibly fresh green sauces, such as the Argentinian Chimichurri that I hadn't heard of as a steak sauce. It has broadened my horizons.

I had never made a hot sauce before and I do enjoy using them. I was a little intimated at first but I realized that they're not difficult to make and the flavor from a homemade hot sauce is simply satisfying.

I've been a big fan of Asian chili oils for quite some time. I've seen them in the stores but most often they're made with soybean or canola oil. I was excited to create a five-spice infused oil, and it didn't last long. I used it in everything!

What to do with these sauces?

They all have quite a flavor kick on their own and would bring out flavors from subtler flavored foods or add that extra dimension. It goes without saying, use them as a finishing sauce and drizzle on top of grilled or smoked meats. Use the green fresh sauces and pesto as a marinade and/or brush on grilling meats and vegetables.

Feel free to experiment.

Scallion Ginger Sauce

One of my favorites, this simple fresh sauce goes well with grilled chicken or pork.

Makes: ½ cup | **Serving Size:** 2 teaspoons

4 scallions, roughly minced (about ⅓ cup)

1-inch ginger root, peeled and roughly minced

1 teaspoon sea salt, divided

3 tablespoons avocado oil

2 bird's-eye chilies, finely minced (optional)

1. Chop the scallions, ginger, and ½ teaspoon salt of together to bring out the juices.

2. Once finely chopped, transfer to a bowl and stir in the avocado oil, remaining sea salt, and chilies, if using.

3. Transfer to a container and let rest for 15 to 30 minutes at room temperature to allow the flavors to combine.

4. It's best when consumed within a day.

NUTRITION PER SERVING: Calories: 32 | **Net Carbohydrates:** 0.2g | **Fat:** 3.5g | **Protein:** 0g | **Carbohydrates:** 0.2g | **Fiber:** 0g

Ale and Pedro's Colombian Aji

This is Ale's hotter take on a savory Colombian condiment. Great over grilled chicken.

Makes: 1 cup | **Serving Size:** 1 teaspoon

10 bird's-eye chilies, chopped

1 medium onion, diced

1 cup chopped parsley

1 cup chopped cilantro

½ cup apple cider vinegar

2 tablespoons extra-virgin olive oil

salt, to taste

black pepper, to taste

1. Mix all of the ingredients together in a small saucepan. Bring to a boil over medium heat for 2 to 3 minutes.

2. Let cool and season with salt and black pepper to taste.

3. Store in the fridge in a glass jar for up to 2 weeks.

NUTRITION PER SERVING: Calories: 6 | **Net Carbohydrates:** 0.3g | **Fat:** 0.4g | **Protein:** 0.1g | **Carbohydrates:** 0.4g | **Fiber:** 0.1g

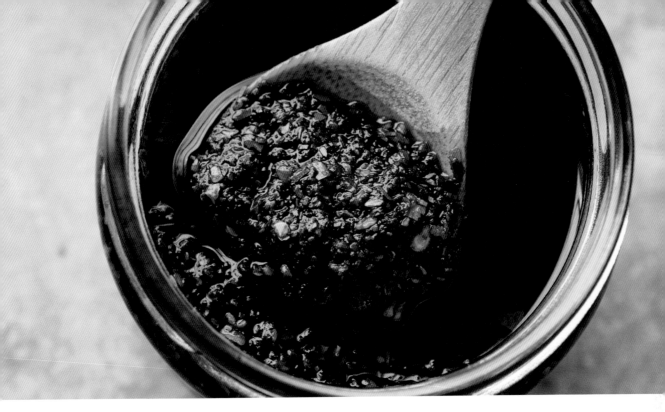

Chili Oil

Brush on this chili oil while grilling zucchini, onion, or mushrooms.

Makes: ⅓ cup | **Serving Size:** 1 teaspoon (includes chili flakes)

⅓ cup avocado oil

2 tablespoons chili flakes

1 teaspoon dried garlic, minced (optional)

1. In a small saucepan over the lowest heat setting, warm the avocado oil and chili flakes, using a thermometer to keep heat them at about 190 to 200°F (88 to 93°C) for approximately 5 minutes.

2. Remove from the heat and let cool to about 180 to185°F (82 to 85°C).

3. Add the dried minced garlic to the pan, if desired.

4. Let cool before transferring to a jar. The oil can be stored on the countertop for a couple of weeks. Stir before using.

NUTRITION PER SERVING: Calories: 42 | **Net Carbohydrates:** 0.2g | **Fat:** 4.7g | **Protein:** 0.1g | **Carbohydrates:** 0.4g | **Fiber:** 0.2g

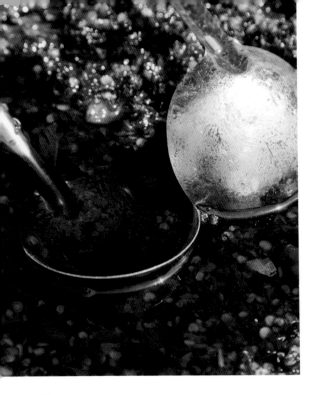

Five-Spice Chili Oil

A drizzled teaspoon of this five-spice chili oil goes a long way! The earthiness of the five spices and the heat of this oil adds another layer of flavor to barbecued meats and grilled vegetables.

Makes: ½ cup | **Serving Size:** 1 teaspoon (includes chili flakes)

½ cup avocado oil

1 teaspoon Sichuan peppercorns

1 teaspoon whole cloves

1 teaspoon whole star anise

1 teaspoon fennel seeds

1-inch cinnamon stick

2 tablespoons chili flakes

1 tablespoon Korean chili flakes

1. In a small saucepan over the lowest heat setting, warm the avocado oil, Sichuan peppercorns, cloves, star anise, fennel seeds, and cinnamon stick for 15 to 20 minutes.

2. There may be a little bubbling but use a thermometer to make sure the temperature is between 230 to 245°F (110 to 118°C). If the temperature rises a little higher, remove the saucepan from the stove temporarily to lower the temperature and avoid burning the spices.

3. After 15 to 20 minutes, remove the saucepan from the heat and wait until the temperature drops to 180 to 185°F (82 to 85°C).

4. Add the chili flakes to a heatproof container, like a canning jar placed on a heatproof surface.

5. Once the oil has reached the desired temperature, very carefully pour the oil through a metal sieve into the jar.

6. Let sit for about 15 to 20 minutes.

7. Stir the chili flakes around in the jar. The chili oil is ready to enjoy. The oil can be stored on the countertop for up to a couple of weeks. Stir the chili oil before using.

NUTRITION PER SERVING: Calories: 42 | **Net Carbohydrates:** 0.2g | **Fat:** 4.7g | **Protein:** 0.1g | **Carbohydrates:** 0.4g | **Fiber:** 0.2g

Three Chili Pepper Hot Sauce

This medium hot sauce is inspired by sriracha hot sauce and goes through a two-week ferment in the fridge. Sriracha hot sauce is traditionally made with red (ripened) jalapeño peppers. I couldn't find any in my area and I tried to ripen them myself without any luck. Enjoy the initial flavors of garlic and chili peppers, followed by a few waves of pleasant heat. Try making it with different chilies.

Makes: 1¼ cups | **Serving Size:** 1 teaspoon

4 serrano chili peppers, 2 each of red and green, roughly chopped

3 jalapeño peppers, roughly chopped

10 bird's-eye peppers, roughly chopped

3 cloves garlic

1 tablespoon apple cider vinegar

1½ teaspoons sea salt

6 tablespoons water, divided

2 tablespoons granular Swerve

1 teaspoon rice vinegar

1. Add all of the chilies, the garlic, apple cider vinegar, salt, and 2 tablespoons of water to a blender.

2. Blend to break down the chilies to the point where the seeds are still intact.

3. Transfer the mash to a glass jar, cover with cheesecloth, and use an elastic band to secure it.

4. Let the chili mash sit on the countertop for a few hours and then place in the fridge for about 2 weeks. It will slightly discolor throughout. If there's mold growth, discard.

5. Transfer the mash to a saucepan and add the Swerve, rice vinegar, and remaining 4 tablespoons of water.

6. Cook over medium heat for about 10 to15 minutes.

7. Turn off the heat and let cool.

8. Transfer to a blender and blend fine. If it's too thick, add water to reach desired consistency. Use caution when opening up the blender jar, don't inhale the vapors.

9. Transfer to a glass container and store in the fridge for 2 to 3 weeks.

NUTRITION PER SERVING: Calories: 2 | **Net Carbohydrates:** 0.4g | **Fat:** 0g | **Protein:** 0.1g | **Carbohydrates:** 0.5g | **Fiber:** 0.1g

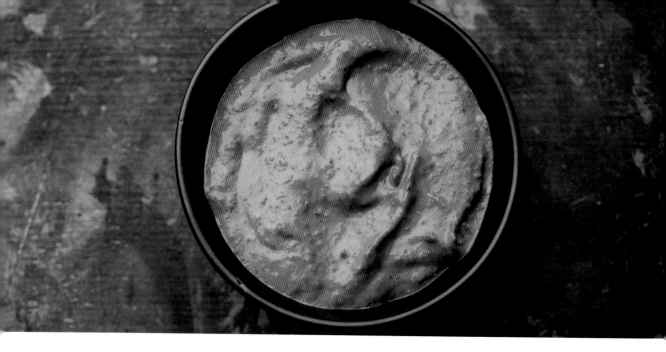

Peri Peri Hot Sauce

A medium-hot, bright citrusy sauce uses peri peri chilies, which are also known as bird's-eye.

Makes: ¾ cup | **Serving Size:** 1 teaspoon

1 tablespoon avocado or olive oil

½ cup onion, chopped

3 cloves garlic, lightly crushed

16 bird's-eye chilies, coarsely chopped

2 tablespoons white vinegar

3 tablespoons lemon juice

1 tablespoon water

½ teaspoon salt

1 teaspoon paprika or smoked paprika

½ teaspoon granular Swerve

¼ teaspoon fish sauce (optional)

1. In a medium saucepan over medium-high heat, add the oil. Once the oil is hot, add the chopped onion and sauté for about 5 minutes, until softened.

2. Add the garlic and quickly sauté for about 15 seconds, until just fragrant.

3. Stir in the remaining ingredients and cook for about a minute or two, then remove from the heat.

4. Let cool, then blend fine in a mixer. If the mixture is too thick, mix in water a tablespoon at a time until the desired consistency is reached.

5. Transfer to a glass jar and cover. Store in the fridge for up to 2 weeks.

NUTRITION PER SERVING: Calories: 6 | **Net Carbohydrates:** 0.5g | **Fat:** 0.4g | **Protein:** 0.1g | **Carbohydrates:** 0.6g | **Fiber:** 0.1g

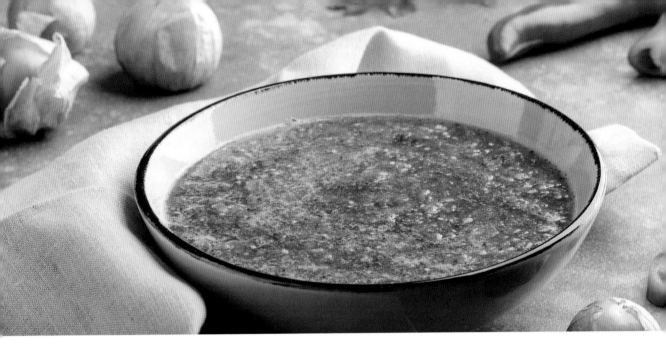

Smoky Chili Verde Sauce

This recipe is great, especially if you've got the grill warmed up and ready to go. This sauce is fabulous with fish tacos and chicken burgers.

Makes: 2½ cups | **Serving Size:** 2 tablespoons

2 poblano peppers

4 jalapeño peppers (fourth pepper is optional; add it halved and raw if some heat is desired)

1 medium onion, halved

5 tomatillos, husks removed

2 cloves garlic

2 teaspoons ground cumin

2 teaspoons dried oregano

juice and zest of 1 lime

2 teaspoons salt

¼ bunch fresh cilantro

1. Place the poblano, jalapeño peppers, onion, and tomatillos on a medium grill. Grill for 2 to 3 minutes, flip over, and grill for an additional 2 minutes or until the desired char is reached.

2. Cut the peppers in half and scrape out seeds. Remove the skin from the onion.

3. Add all of the ingredients to a food processor and blend until uniform.

4. The sauce is ready to use. Store in the fridge in a glass container for up to 1 week.

NUTRITION PER SERVING: **Calories:** 12 | **Net Carbohydrates:** 1.7g | **Fat:** 0.2g | **Protein:** 0.4g | **Carbohydrates:** 2.5g | **Fiber:** 0.8g

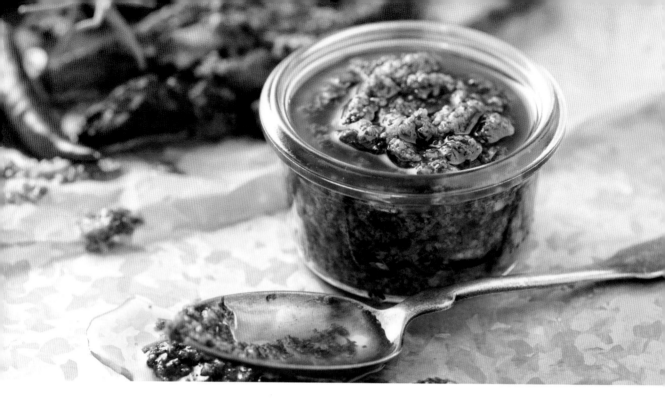

Chimichurri

This uncooked sauce originates in Argentina. A fresh, vibrant, versatile sauce used in cooking or marinating, it's best served with grilled steak.

Makes: 1¼ cups | **Serving Size:** 1 tablespoon

1 cup coarsely chopped flat leaf parsley

½ cup coarsely chopped cilantro

1 to 2 cloves garlic, coarsely chopped

1 teaspoon Mexican dried oregano

1 to 2 bird's-eye chilies, chopped fine

2 tablespoons apple cider vinegar

2 tablespoons lemon juice

½ cup extra-virgin olive oil

1 teaspoon salt

1. Chop the flat-leaf parsley, cilantro, and garlic together with a knife. Once they have reached a fine consistency, add them to a medium bowl and mix in the rest of the ingredients.

2. Cover and let the chimichurri rest in the fridge for a few hours, or better yet overnight, for the flavors to develop.

3. Store in a covered container in the fridge for 2 to 3 days.

NUTRITION PER SERVING: Calories: 51 | **Net Carbohydrates:** 0.3g |
Fat: 5.7g | **Protein:** 0.2g | **Carbohydrates:** 0.5g | **Fiber:** 0.2g

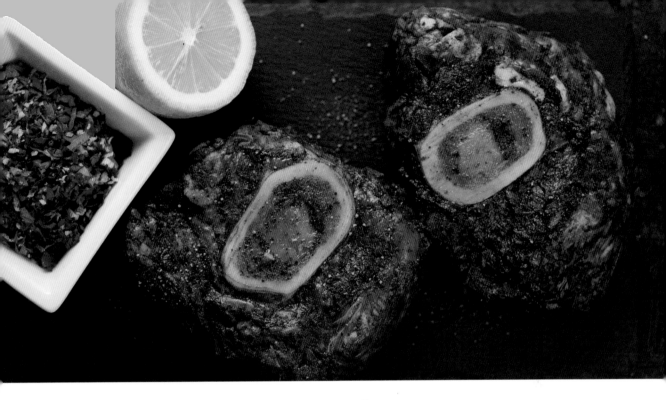

Gremolata

This traditional fresh Italian green condiment pairs really well with a
nice grilled steak. Or, use it as a marinade with a citrus kick.

Makes: about ½ cup | **Serving Size:** 1 teaspoon

1½ cups roughly chopped Italian flat
leafed parsley (about 1 bunch)

2 to 3 cloves garlic, minced

5 tablespoons lemon juice

zest from 1 lemon

salt, to taste

splash of white vinegar

1. Chop garlic and parsley together to fine pieces.

2. Transfer the chopped garlic and parsley to a small bowl and mix in the lemon juice,
lemon zest, and salt.

3. Cover and let the flavors marinate in the fridge for an hour.

4. Store covered in the fridge for 2 to 3 days.

NUTRITION PER SERVING: **Calories:** 5 | **Net Carbohydrates:** 1.0g |
Fat: 0.1g | **Protein:** 0.2g | **Carbohydrates:** 1.2g | **Fiber:** 0.2g

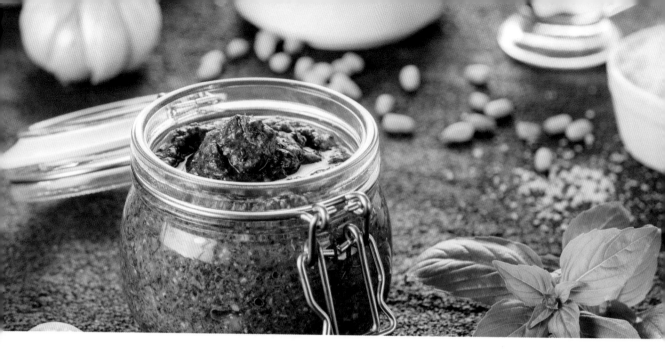

Basic Pesto

It's always nice to have fresh pesto on hand for so many uses. Drizzle it on grilled vegetables or mix it in with mayonnaise for an aioli. Use it as a marinade with chicken or fish.

Try adding some variation by substituting out basil with parsley, kale, or cilantro. Add more fats by using macadamia or pili nuts instead of pine nuts.

Makes: ¾ cup | **Serving Size:** 1 tablespoon

2 cups fresh basil leaves

2 tablespoons toasted pine nuts

2 to 3 cloves garlic

¼ cup grated Parmesan cheese

¼ cup extra-virgin olive oil

1. Add all of the ingredients to a food processor or blender and blend until everything is uniform.

2. Use immediately or store in the fridge, noting that the pesto will become solid when kept in the fridge. Pull it out 10 minutes before using for the olive oil to become liquid again, then stir to mix.

3. Store covered in the fridge for up to 1 week.

> **NUTRITION PER SERVING: Calories:** 64 | **Net Carbohydrates:** 0.5g |
> **Fat:** 6.7g | **Protein:** 1.1g | **Carbohydrates:** 0.8g | **Fiber:** 0.3g

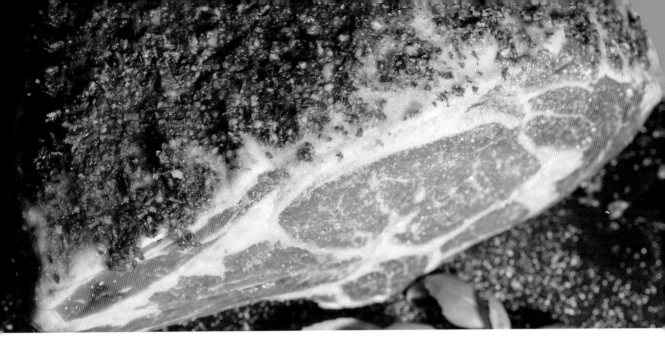

Pili Nut Pesto

Pili nuts are a creamier and fattier nut with a very low carb count compared to other nuts. Adding coconut oil elevates this pesto even further to bring in those healthy good fats. No guilt here. Add that extra spoonful to top off that steak!

Makes: ½ cup | **Serving Size:** 1 tablespoon

½ cup packed fresh basil

½ cup packed fresh cilantro

1 clove garlic, crushed

¼ cup powdered Parmesan cheese

¼ cup pili nuts

½ teaspoon salt

2 tablespoons extra-virgin olive oil

2 tablespoons liquid coconut oil

1. Place the basil, cilantro, garlic, parmesan cheese, pili nuts, and salt in a food processor and pulse until mixed and crumbly.

2. Add the oils and blend until creamy.

3. Let rest for 15 minutes to infuse the flavors.

4. Use immediately or store in the fridge, noting that the pesto will become solid when kept in the fridge. Pull it out 10 minutes before using for the olive oil/coconut oil to become liquid again, then stir to mix.

5. Store in the fridge in a covered container for up to 7 days.

NUTRITION PER SERVING: **Calories:** 77 | **Net Carbohydrates:** 0.8g | **Fat:** 7.4g | **Protein:** 2.9g | **Carbohydrates:** 0.9g | **Fiber:** 0.1g

CHAPTER 10

Relishes and More

A relish refers to a condiment that's cooked and then pickled, usually consisting of a mix of fruits, vegetables, herbs, and spices.

Most often the pickling process involves water bath canning along with a copious amount of sugar, salt, and vinegar. I'm not sure how the canning process or food safety would be affected by substituting the sugar with a sweetener, so I thought it would be best to avoid canning all together.

These are really chunky condiments to serve a couple of tablespoons of on the side or on top of a burger, jumbo hot dog, or grilled or smoked meats. More often than not, you'll find yourself looking for something to scoop (a pork rind perhaps?) these tasty condiments up and eat them like a dip!

Bacon Jam

Warning: This may never make it to the table! A savory, smoky condiment with bacon, this jam will bring those burgers (or anything!) to a whole new level.

Makes: 1 cup | Serving Size: 1 tablespoon

½ pound bacon ends, cubed

pinch of salt

1 cup julienned onion

2 tablespoons water

2 tablespoons brown Swerve

¼ teaspoon ground cinnamon

¼ teaspoon chipotle chili powder

¼ teaspoon salt

⅓ cup water

2 tablespoons apple cider vinegar

1 tablespoon butter

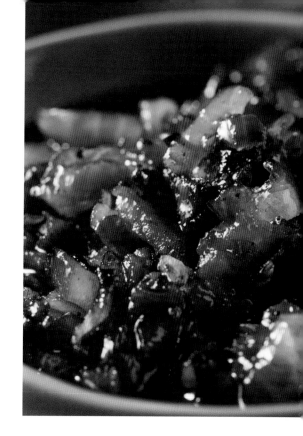

1. In a medium skillet over medium heat, cook the bacon ends with a pinch of salt. Sauté for 5 to 6 minutes. Remove the bacon ends from pan and set aside, keeping heat on medium.

2. Add the onion to the bacon grease in the same skillet, along with 2 teaspoons of water, stirring occasionally. Allow the onions to soften and caramelize slightly, about 5 minutes.

3. In a small bowl, mix the brown Swerve, cinnamon, chipotle chili powder, and salt. Set aside.

4. Add the ¼ teaspoon of water, apple cider vinegar, and butter to the skillet with the onion.

5. Mix in the spice mix and turn the heat down to low.

6. Simmer, uncovered, to reduce the liquid, stirring occasionally for 20 minutes.

7. Once the mixture has reached a thick jam–like consistency, remove from the heat and let cool.

8. Transfer to a covered glass jar and store in the fridge for up to a week.

NUTRITION PER SERVING: Calories: 69 | **Net Carbohydrates:** 0.7g | **Fat:** 6.4g | **Protein:** 1.9g | **Carbohydrates:** 0.9g | **Fiber:** 0.2g

Strawberry Relish

Look out burgers and grilled chicken! Here comes a savory and tangy relish with a hint of strawberries that salutes summer.

Makes: 1¼ cups | **Serving Size:** 1 tablespoon

1 cup chopped tomatoes

½ cup finely chopped strawberries

1 tablespoon chopped fresh basil

1 tablespoon apple cider vinegar

1 teaspoon balsamic vinegar

¼ cup finely chopped red onion

½ teaspoon cracked coriander seed

¼ teaspoon confectioner's Swerve

¼ teaspoon sea salt

¼ teaspoon black pepper

½ teaspoon red chili flakes (optional)

1. Mix all of the ingredients together in a medium bowl.

2. Cover and refrigerate for at least a couple of hours, but overnight is best.

3. Store in the fridge in a covered container for up to 3 days.

NUTRITION PER SERVING: Calories: 4 | **Net Carbohydrates:** 0.8g | **Fat:** 0g | **Protein:** 0.1g | **Carbohydrates:** 1.0g | **Fiber:** 0.2g

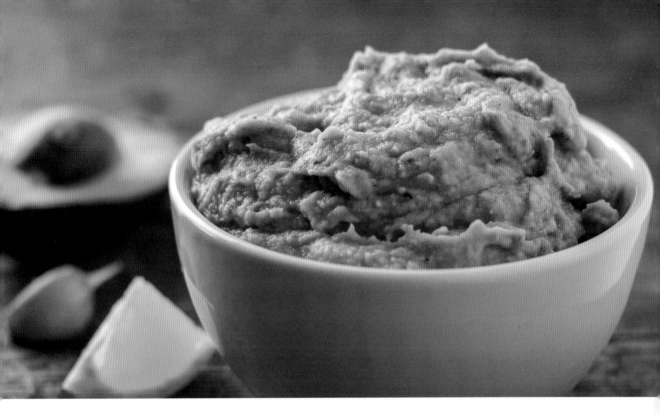

Guacamole

This is a guacamole where less is more. It is a very flavorful condiment that is packed with all the beneficial fats, electrolytes, and vitamins from the avocado fruit. It's absolutely fantastic on burgers. Give it a go the next time you have brisket.

Makes: ½ cup | **Serving Size:** 2 tablespoons

1 medium avocado, roughly chopped

1½ tablespoons lime juice

½ teaspoon sea salt

1 tablespoon chopped fresh cilantro

1. Mash the avocado in a mortar and pestle or in a bowl using a fork.

2. Add the mashed avocado, lime juice, and the sea salt to a bowl, and mash.

3. Mix in the chopped cilantro.

4. The guacamole is ready to use and best when made fresh.

NUTRITION PER SERVING: Calories: 41 | **Net Carbohydrates:** 0.9g | **Fat:** 3.7g | **Protein:** 0.5g | **Carbohydrates:** 2.6g | **Fiber:** 1.7g

Spicy Guacamole

What a way to get those good fats in style! Flavorful enough but not too spicy, it still imparts that avocado flavor. Try it with chicken grilled using the Tex–Mex Rub (page 44).

Makes: 1½ cups | **Serving Size:** 1 tablespoon

1 teaspoon ancho chili powder

1 teaspoon dried Mexican oregano

1 teaspoon paprika

¼ teaspoon ground cumin

¼ teaspoon ground cayenne pepper

½ teaspoon sea salt

¼ teaspoon coarsely cracked black peppercorns

3 medium avocados, mashed

1 tablespoon full–fat sour cream

2 tablespoons chopped pickled jalapeños

2 tablespoons lime juice

2 teaspoons lime zest

½ teaspoon hot sauce (optional)

2 tablespoons chopped fresh cilantro

1. Mix the spices together in a small bowl and set aside.

2. Mix the wet ingredients together in a separate bowl.

3. Stir the spice mix into the wet ingredients.

4. Cover and place in the fridge for an hour before serving.

5. Best when it's made fresh, but it can be stored in a covered container and consumed within a couple of days.

NUTRITION PER SERVING: **Calories:** 23 | **Net Carbohydrates:** 0.5g | **Fat:** 2g | **Protein:** 0.3g | **Carbohydrates:** 1.5g | **Fiber:** 1.0g

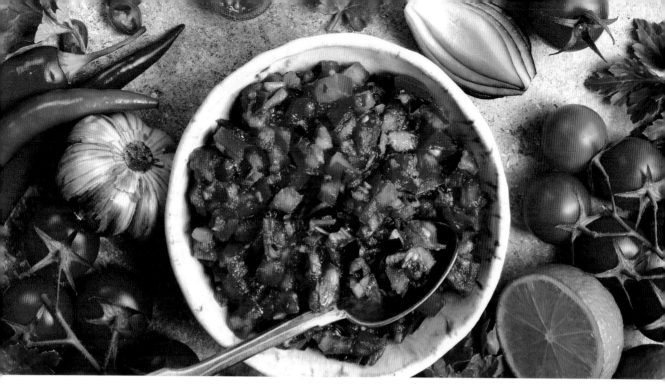

Pico de Gallo

A fresh salsa that brings those vibrant flavors to the barbecue for you to celebrate summer—or any season—with friends. For something a little different, char the onion, jalapeño, and half the tomatoes on the grill before chopping.

Makes: 3½ cups | Serving Size: 1 tablespoon

3 large tomatoes, chopped fine

½ medium red onion, chopped

1 jalapeño pepper, chopped

1½ teaspoons ground cumin

2 teaspoons sea salt

2 tablespoons lime juice

2 teaspoons lime zest

½ bunch chopped fresh cilantro

1. Mix all the ingredients together in a large bowl.

2. Cover and place in the fridge for a couple of hours to infuse the flavors before serving.

3. Store in the fridge in a covered container. Pico de Gallo is best when eaten within a couple of days.

NUTRITION PER SERVING: **Calories:** 5 | **Net Carbohydrates:** 0.7g | **Fat:** 0.1g | **Protein:** 0.2g | **Carbohydrates:** 1g | **Fiber:** 0.3g

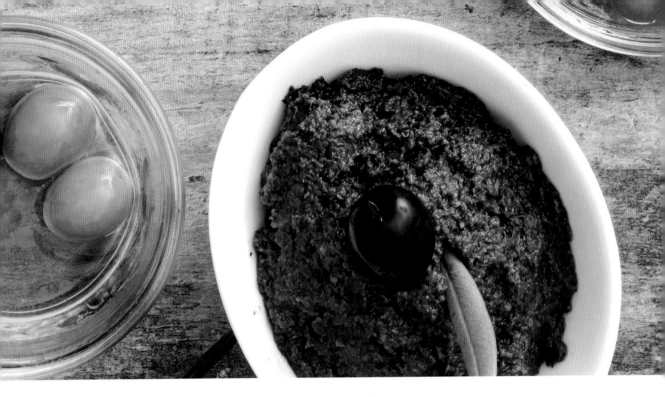

Tapenade

An umami-packed, chunky condiment to serve alongside vegetables, chicken, and lamb.

Makes: 1¼ cups | **Serving Size:** 2 tablespoons

½ cup pimento-stuffed olives

½ cup pitted kalamata olives

4 teaspoons lemon juice

2 tablespoons extra-virgin olive oil

2 tablespoons capers, drained

2 cloves garlic

pinch of confectioner's Swerve

2 turns coarsely ground black peppercorns

3 tablespoons chopped fresh cilantro

2 tablespoons chopped fresh basil

½ teaspoon anchovy paste (optional)

1. Place all of the ingredients in a food processor and pulse until all of the ingredients are mixed well and a fine, slightly chunky consistency is reached.

3. Let sit for 30 minutes at room temperature to infuse flavors before serving.

4. Store in the fridge in a covered glass container for up to 2 weeks, noting that the tapenade may become solid when kept in the fridge. Pull it out 10 minutes before using for the olive oil to become liquid again, then stir to mix.

NUTRITION PER SERVING: **Calories:** 26 | **Net Carbohydrates:** 0.3g | **Fat:** 2.7g | **Protein:** 0.2g | **Carbohydrates:** 0.7g | **Fiber:** 0.4g

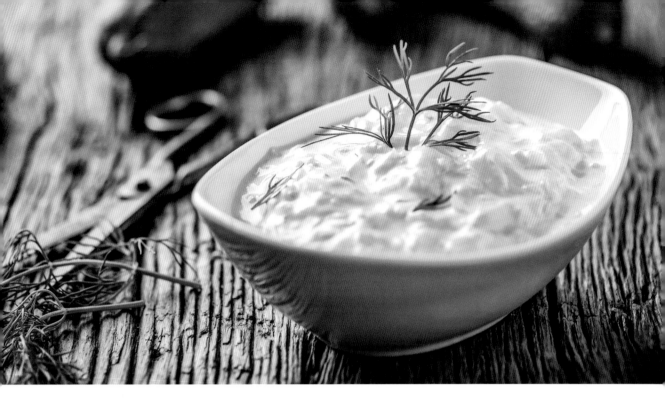

Tzatziki

Instead of yogurt, break out the sour cream. The increased fat gives this tzatziki a richer flavor and mouthfeel. Great to serve with herbaceous flavors but goes well with hot foods to give a little relief. Fabulous with grilled skewers made with the Citrus Marinade (page 49).

Makes: 1 cup | **Serving Size:** 1 tablespoon

½ cup grated cucumber, seeds removed

½ tablespoon dried dill

1 tablespoon lemon juice

1 to 2 cloves garlic, crushed

1 cup full-fat sour cream

1 teaspoon sea salt

¼ teaspoon black pepper

1. Squeeze the grated cucumber in a clean kitchen or paper towel to remove some of the water.

2. Add the cucumber to a medium bowl and mix in the remaining ingredients. Refrigerate for a couple of hours before serving.

3. Store in the fridge in a covered glass or plastic container and consume within 3 to 4 days.

NUTRITION PER SERVING: Calories: 30 | **Net Carbohydrates:** 1.0g | **Fat:** 2.8 | **Protein:** 0.4g | **Carbohydrates:** 1.1g | **Fiber:** 0.1g

Zucchini Relish

A sweet and tangy relish to accompany those smokies, hot dogs, and burgers. Make it the day before to let the flavors develop.

Makes: 2 cups | **Serving Size:** 2 tablespoons

2 cups grated cucumber, seeds removed

3 cups grated zucchini, seeds removed

1 tablespoon sea salt

¼ cup apple cider vinegar

⅓ cup white vinegar

1/16 teaspoon ground turmeric

⅓ cup granular Swerve

¾ teaspoon mustard seeds

½ teaspoon crushed chili flakes

½ teaspoon dried dill (optional)

½ teaspoon cracked coriander seed

¼ teaspoon celery seeds

2 tablespoons brown Swerve

½ medium onion, chopped

1 clove garlic, finely minced

1. Place the grated cucumber in a clean kitchen or paper towel and squeeze out the water. Remove from the towel and place the cucumber in a strainer to let any residual water drain.

2. Repeat with the grated zucchini.

3. In a bowl, massage the sea salt into both the zucchini and cucumber. Let sit for an hour.

4. In a saucepan over low heat, warm the vinegars for about 5 minutes.

5. Add the spices to the vinegars, and whisk in the sweetener. Continue heating for another 5 minutes or until the sweetener is dissolved.

6. Mix the onion and garlic with the spiced vinegar. Turn off the heat.

7. Add the zucchini and cucumber to the saucepan and mix well. Make sure that all the vegetable is coated with the vinegar.

8. Transfer the mixture to a canning jar or a bowl, and cover.

9. Place in the fridge and let rest for 24 hours before diving in.

10. Store in a covered jar in the fridge for up to a week.

NUTRITION PER SERVING: Calories: 14 | **Net Carbohydrates:** 1.8g | **Fat:** 0.2g | **Protein:** 1.0g | **Carbohydrates:** 2.4g | **Fiber:** 0.6g

Conversions

Volume

U.S.	U.S. Equivalent	Metric
1 tablespoon (3 teaspoons)	½ fluid ounce	15 milliliters
¼ cup	2 fluid ounces	60 milliliters
⅓ cup	3 fluid ounces	90 milliliters
½ cup	4 fluid ounces	120 milliliters
⅔ cup	5 fluid ounces	150 milliliters
¾ cup	6 fluid ounces	180 milliliters
1 cup	8 fluid ounces	240 milliliters
2 cups	16 fluid ounces	480 milliliters

Weight

U.S.	Metric
½ ounce	15 grams
1 ounce	30 grams
2 ounces	60 grams
¼ pound	115 grams
⅓ pound	150 grams
½ pound	225 grams
¾ pound	350 grams
1 pound	450 grams

Temperature

Fahrenheit (°F)	Celsius (°C)
70°F	20°C
100°F	40°C
120°F	50°C
130°F	55°C
140°F	60°C
150°F	65°C
160°F	70°C
170°F	75°C
180°F	80°C
190°F	90°C
200°F	95°C

Fahrenheit (°F)	Celsius (°C)
220°F	105°C
240°F	115°C
260°F	125°C
280°F	140°C
300°F	150°C
325°F	165°C
350°F	175°C
375°F	190°C
400°F	200°C
425°F	220°C
450°F	230°C

Acknowledgments

I am ever so thankful for all the people that have supported me throughout this project. Whether through words of encouragement, feedback on recipes, or plying me with caffeine, I'm grateful to have you!

Thank you to the phenomenal crew at Ulysses Press for having me jump on another fun and crazy ride. Many, many thanks to all the people behind the scenes who helped put this project together.

To my husband, Jeffrey, for surviving the tornado of kitchen activity and just for being there for me.

To the revived taste-testing crew at UFV, thank you for letting me hear your thoughts on my cooking once again, and for your never-ending support!

To my Starbucks Salish Plaza family, thank you for keeping my coffee mug full and allowing me to take up residence in the corner. I'm so happy you had a chance to taste a few of these!

A special thank you to Gord and Jane Webb for sharing their Blueberry Barbecue Sauce recipe and to Alexandra and Pedro Montoya-Pelaez for sharing their Colombian Aji recipe, who were excited to hear about this project. Both couples were eager to share their love for barbecue by sharing a few of their favorite recipes.

About the Author

Five years ago, **Aileen Ablog** discovered the ketogenic diet when she was faced with a future of health ailments. She needed to lose weight and changed her eating habits. Within a few months of weight loss and increased energy, she realized this was more than just a diet; it became a lifestyle.

She lives in Chilliwack, BC, with her husband, Jeffrey, and their feisty cat, Bessie. By day she works at the University of the Fraser Valley as a chemistry lab technician. Rumor has it, she can also be seen behind the counter at Starbucks working on her latte art. She enjoys cooking, watching movies, and drinking coffee.